A RADIOGRAPHER'S HANDBOOK OF HOSPITAL PRACTICE

The authors wish to dedicate this little handbook to all their students over many years and to those who come afterwards.

A Radiographer's Handbook of Hospital Practice

D. Noreen Chesney FCR, TE
Muriel O. Chesney FCR, TE

BLACKWELL SCIENTIFIC PUBLICATIONS
OXFORD LONDON EDINBURGH
BOSTON PALO ALTO MELBOURNE

Editorial offices:
Osney Mead, Oxford, OX2 OEL
8 John Street, London, WC1N 2ES
23 Ainslie Place, Edinburgh, EH3 6AJ
52 Beacon Street, Boston, Massachusetts 02108, USA
667 Lytton Avenue, Palo Alto, California 94301, USA
107 Barry Street, Carlton, Victoria 3053, Australia

First published 1986

Set by Katerprint Typesetting Services, Oxford
Printed in Great Britain by Billing & Sons Ltd, Worcester

DISTRIBUTORS

USA
Blackwell Mosby Book Distributors
11830 Westline Industrial Drive
St Louis, Missouri 63141

Canada
The C.V. Mosby Company
5240 Finch Avenue East,
Scarborough, Ontario

Australia
Blackwell Scientific Publications (Australia) Pty Ltd
107 Barry Street
Carlton, Victoria 3053

British Library
Cataloguing in Publication Data

Chesney, D. Noreen
A radiographer's handbook of hospital practice.
1. Diagnosis, Radioscopic
I. Title II. Chesney, Muriel O.
616.07'57'024613 RC78

ISBN 0-632-01487-3

Contents

Preface, vii
1 First contact with a patient, 1
2 Principles in lifting and moving patients, 3
3 The use of drugs and agents, 7
4 Giving bedpans and urinals, 10
5 Taking the radial pulse, 13
6 Taking the oral temperature, 15
7 Counting the respiration, 17
8 Recording the blood pressure, 18
9 Procedure for giving an enema, 20
10 Laying up a sterile trolley, 22
11 Technique for a simple sterile dressing, 24
12 Assisting with an intravenous injection, 28
13 The use of oxygen, 32
14 Care before, during and after general anaesthesia, 35
15 Accidents and dangerous occurrences, 38
16 Actions in the event of a fire, 42
17 Radiological emergencies, 44
18 Some first aid, 47
19 An infectious patient in the ward, 74
20 An infectious patient in the X-ray department, 76
21 The patient with a tracheostomy, 78
22 Tracheo-bronchial suction, 80
23 The patient with a colostomy/ileostomy, 84
24 The ten-day rule, 86

25 General abdominal preparation, 90
26 Barium meal, 92
27 Barium enema, 94
28 Intravenous urogram, 96
29 Oral cholecystogram, 99
30 Intravenous cholangiography, 101
31 Bronchography, 104
32 Hysterosalpingography, 107
33 Angiography, 109
34 Lymphangiography, 113
35 Radiculography/myelography, 118
36 CT scans, 123
37 Medical ultrasound, 125
38 Radionuclide imaging, 127
Index, 131

Preface

We have written this handbook mainly for one group of readers whose needs have been lodged firmly in our minds for many years: student radiographers. In writing it, we have sought to provide a book which might be: small and handy to use; not so costly as to make you too hesitant to buy it; a ready source of information for answering practical queries or for revision.

We hope that we have succeeded in implementing our intentions. As to the material selected to make the book, we have been significantly influenced by the contents of two other publications. These are, firstly, Chesney and Chesney's *Care of the Patient in Diagnostic Radiography*, to which we would refer the readers of this handbook for fuller dissertations on these matters. Secondly, we have had regard to the syllabus of training of the College of Radiographers in the United Kingdom and those sections in it which relate to hospital practice and care of the patient as determining what the students are required to know.

We would like here to express a word of thanks to a teacher: Miss A.F. Shaw, Principal (Radiotherapy), The Central Birmingham School of Radiography, who freely gave one of us the help of some personal discussion about radionuclide imaging.

In conclusion, we wish all of you (teachers and students alike) the best of luck.

D.N.C.
M.O.C.

Chapter 1

First contact with a patient

1 You must be ready. Readiness implies consideration of the following factors:

(a) the department as a whole;

(b) the X-ray room and all items of equipment and accessories which are to be used for the procedure;

(c) yourself as a professional radiographer, having regard to your appearance, your personal hygiene, your behaviour and your attitude of mind.

2 Check the request form for the examination and make sure that you know what is to be done, to whom it is to be done and for what reasons it is to be done.

3 Greet the patient and make him welcome.

4 Positively identify the patient with reference to:

(a) name, age, address;

(b) hospital number;

(c) notes and any previous radiographs and reports;

(d) his hospital identity bracelet if he is wearing one.

5 Explain to the patient what is to be done and give him clear but not intimidating instructions so that he knows what he must do.

6 While you talk to him, mentally assess and review the situation and the radiographic procedure to be undertaken. You should find yourself considering the following points:

(a) the condition of the patient;

(b) the existence of special features of the patient which may call for special care;
(c) the radiographic procedures;
(d) any predictable difficulties in carrying out the procedure which become apparent now that you have met the patient;
(e) any solutions to specific problems.

7 Escort the patient to the X-ray room.

8 Throughout the time that you are with the patient, observe him, listen to him and care about him, remembering that attention to detail distinguishes between those who think and those who do not.

9 After the procedure is over, see the patient safely away. He should be left with a pleasant impression of you as a radiographer and he should know of any special instructions or advice that he must follow.

Chapter 2

Principles in lifting and moving patients

When you lift a patient the transfer should be smooth, unalarming and safe not only for the patient but also for yourself. If you cannot achieve this in regard to yourself, you will be less likely to achieve it for the patient.

It is important for the lifter to achieve balance and so you must:

(a) consider your centre of gravity, which in the erect human body is at the level of the second sacral vertebra;

(b) consider your base, which is that area over which your body is supported as you stand on the ground;

(c) realize that if your line of gravity (a vertical line which passes through the centre of gravity) meets the ground within your base, you are balanced and will not fall over;

(d) realize that the larger is your base the greater is your stability;

(e) realize that your standing base can be enlarged by keeping your feet apart, since with your feet separated your base becomes the area of ground covered by your feet, extended by the area of the space between them.

By now you will probably have found that when you want to achieve a stable balance for a special effort you unconsciously seek this stability by moving your feet apart. You will spread your feet in one or the other of two ways:

(a) by placing the feet apart side by side and parallel as if straddling an invisible object (an imaginary bicycle?);
(b) by placing the feet apart one in front of the other as if in a frozen walking step.

In order to help you to lift safely, we set out below some important imperatives which embody the basic principles of successful lifting.

1 *Prepare to lift.*

In this preparation you review the space available, where the patient now is and where you want him eventually to be. You consider the placings of lifters. You plan the most economic expenditure of energy: for example, you ensure that the distance through which the patient has to be lifted and moved is as short as is practicable.

2 *Choose the type of lift to be used.*

In making the choice, you have certain questions in your mind. What is the lifting to be done? Is it a patient from a wheelchair to an X-ray table? What help can the patient give? How many people will lift? You must make sure that you do have enough people for the task.

3 *Position the lifters carefully.*

In positioning the lifters, the important points are the proximity of the lifters to the patient and the postures and the stances of the lifters. Poor access to the patient, so that the lifter is unable to assume freely the most favourable posture and stance and an attempt to lift a load from a position too far away are both likely causes of some damage to the lifter; perhaps also of damage to the load and certainly of some uneasiness of any load who is a conscious human being.

4 *Remember always the most favourable stance and posture.*

To achieve these you need to have the following considerations in mind.

(a) Your feet must be apart to broaden your base.

(b) You *must* protect your back from injury by using your strong leg muscles to take the strain of the load. You make use of your legs by flexing at hips and knees and ankles *before* you lift and then straightening at these joints *during* the lift. You do not bend your back at all. If the load is at a low level, get down to the required nearness to it by bending your legs to squat with your back kept straight. Maintain your back as straight as you can while you lift and carry a heavy load. You can keep your spine held straight by the action of abdominal bracing: contract your lower abdomen with an action that is directed up towards the waist and outwards from the mid-line towards the sides of the trunk. As you perform this abdominal brace, stretch your back and raise your head a little and you should find that your whole body has been given firmness and security to maintain the posture of a straight back as you lift.

(c) You can more easily support a load which you are carrying if you hold it close to your trunk by bending your elbows and keeping your upper arms close to your body.

5 *Consider the grasps to be used.*

The point to remember here is that a broader gripping surface gives more security of hold.

6 Remember that 'the team' must apply their forces and act for the transfer and the lift *together*.

The team may be:

(a) one lifter (you) and the patient, in which case you are the person directing the transfer;

(b) two or more lifters and the patient, in which case one of the lifters must be designated as the director of the transfer or lift. To achieve optimum coordination, the director should ensure that everyone (and that includes a conscious patient) is fully instructed as to what is going to be done and all know what action (or perhaps for the patient what maintained lack of action) is individually required of them. Only the director of the lift issues the commands which are needed and it is clearly important that these commands are agreed and are correctly related to the actions to be taken on the commands. To achieve clarity, it is better to use words: get ready, brace yourselves, lift, turn, walk, lower, let go. Counting one, two, three and so on can leave everyone uncertain as to what they should do and at what moments they must act.

Chapter 3

The use of drugs and agents

Categorization

If you visit a hospital pharmacy you will find that there are four particularly important classifications of drugs. These four categories refer to the availability of drugs and each classification imposes further restrictions on the handling and dispensing of the listed drugs. The four categories are as follows.

1 *General Sales List (GSL).*

This list comprises medicines which can be bought and sold in any shop anywhere.

2 *Pharmacy Medicines (P).*

This list contains medicines which can be obtained only in a pharmacy or a chemist's shop where there is a qualified pharmacist on the premises at the time.

3 *Prescription Only Medicines (POM).*

This list has drugs which are obtainable only through a written prescription from a doctor or dentist.

4 *Controlled Drugs (CD).*

The agents on this list are obtainable only on a written prescription from a doctor or dentist with the further restrictions that this be written in the handwriting of the prescriber and that the quantities it mentions must be denoted both in numerals and in words.

Administration of drugs

The following are the main routes of administration of various drugs, medicines and agents which may be given to patients for the purposes of diagnosis or treatment.

1 *Oral administration.*

The patient takes the agent by mouth. This is of course simple and convenient for the patient and is very often used, being regarded as the method of choice unless there is some reason which makes imperative the use of another route.

2 *Parenteral administration.*

Parenteral administration means that the agent is injected by using a hypodermic needle and a syringe. The injection may be:

(a) subcutaneous (just under the skin) if a small amount is given;

(b) intramuscular (into a muscle in the upper arm, the outer aspect of the thigh, the upper outer quadrant of the buttock) if the amount is greater or more rapid absorption is required;

(c) intravenous (into a vein, usually in the arm) if large amounts are to be given and very rapid absorption is required.

3 *Rectal administration.*

In rectal administration the agent is embodied in a solution which is given as an enema or in the solid form of a suppository which is inserted in the rectum.

4 *Inhalation.*

Inhalation is the method of administration for anaesthetic gases.

5 *Local application.*

Drops which are instilled into the eye, the ear or the nose and ointments and lotions which are applied to the skin are examples of local application.

Safe routines

It is most important that you should practise a routine which is meticulously observed and is planned to reduce the chances of error whenever you are called upon to administer any drug or agent to a patient who is in your care. The word care has many meanings and in this context several are apt. You must care in the sense of being concerned; you must care in the sense of providing the patient with protection; you must act with care in the sense of paying serious and sustained attention to what you do. Consider the imperatives below.

1 Make sure that you know with complete certainty:
- (a) to whom the agent is to be given;
- (b) what agent you are to give;
- (c) in what quantity it is to be given;
- (d) how it is to be given;
- (e) when it is to be given.

2 In making any preparations and in giving the agent, make sure that the lighting is good and that you can clearly see what you are doing.

3 Check the labels carefully and be absolutely certain as to the information they contain.

4 Measure amounts accurately and with care.

5 Identify the patient with certainty.

6 Check that the agent has not been previously given by someone else.

7 Observe the rules for a sterile procedure if they apply.

8 Make sure that you give the correct agent in the prescribed amount to the right patient, at the right time, in the right way.

9 If it is required, record appropriately the administration of the agent.

10 If you are assisting a doctor who is giving an intravenous injection remember that you still have responsibility for the items **1** to **7** above.

Chapter 4

Giving bedpans and urinals

The present practice in hospital tries to spare patients the use of bedpans and urinals and encourages a mobility which is as extended as possible: many patients today are allowed to go to the lavatory or to use a commode at the bedside who in earlier years would have been kept fast in bed. Despite this, from time to time a radiographer may have to provide a patient with a bedpan or urinal and so it seemed worthwhile to include here some points on their use.

Giving a bedpan

1 Ensure privacy for the patient.
2 If you can, wear a disposable plastic apron and discard it after use. If you must leave your uniform unprotected with an apron, then you should handle the bedpan carefully to keep your clothes uncontaminated by contact with it.
3 Make sure that the bedpan is warm and dry and that you have a cover for it (for example, a disposable paper sheet) as you take it to the patient.
4 If the patient can raise himself, stand to one side of him (usually the right) and as he lifts slide the bedpan under his buttocks. Avoid scraping him with the bedpan as you do this and make sure that it is the right way round (narrow end to the front) and is in the right place. If the patient can do little to help himself,

so long as you are sure that you can manage alone you should position yourself to one side and place one hand under the lower part of the patient's back. Then raise the patient's buttocks with that hand sufficiently to allow you to use the other hand to slide the bedpan into position. In such circumstances you must be especially careful not to scrape the patient's skin. If the patient is entirely helpless, then you must have an assistant positioned on the opposite side of the patient. You can then command three hands for lifting and one for placing the bedpan. A very heavy patient may need a force of three people to provide four hands for lifting (two from each side) and two hands for placing the bedpan.

5 Make sure that the patient is secure, is appropriately propped up if necessary and feels reasonably easy. We do not think that it is possible to make anyone feel wholly comfortable on a bedpan but you must do your best to ensure that all is as well as it can be.

6 Before you leave the patient, make certain that he knows how to call you back and for yourself make sure that you are available to be called and can reach the patient quickly.

7 Supply toilet paper so that the patient can clean himself: if he cannot manage this, then you must do it for him. Afterwards provide him with the means to wash and dry his hands.

8 Leave the patient comfortable and tidy.

9 Deal with the bedpan appropriately. If it is disposable, macerate it and wash the outer shell. If it is not disposable, put it in the bedpan flush washer and return it clean to the place where it is regularly kept ready for use.

10 Wash and dry your hands.

Giving a urinal

1 Ensure privacy for the patient.

2 Protect your uniform with a plastic apron if you can and discard the apron after use. If no apron is worn, be careful to keep your uniform uncontaminated.

3 Take the urinal covered to the patient.

4 Make sure that he is able to place it for himself to use it and that he can call you back when he has finished.

5 Afterwards see that the patient is comfortable and tidy.

6 Empty the urinal immediately after use and ensure that it is cleaned, disinfected or sterilized and placed upside down to drain. Some urinals are disposable and can, of course, be macerated immediately after use.

Chapter 5

Taking the radial pulse

1 Make sure that you have a watch which indicates seconds of time.
2 The patient should be in a position of rest, either sitting or lying down.
3 Explain to the patient what you are about to do.
4 Flex the patient's forearm (right or left, whichever you propose to use) across his chest with the palm of his hand downwards.
5 If you aim for the patient's right wrist for pulse-counting, be prepared to use the fingers of your left hand for the action and to hold your watch in your right hand. That is, you use the fingers of your hand which is the opposite one to the patient's wrist where you are to count the pulse: your left for his right and your right for his left.
6 Place your first three fingers of the appropriate hand on the patient's wrist firmly along the line of the radial artery (palmar aspect of the wrist on the radial side), resting your thumb on the dorsal aspect of the wrist: the V shape that is formed by the metacarpals of your thumb and index finger should straddle the patient's wrist.
7 When you can detect the beat of the radial pulse with your fingers begin to count it.
8 Count for a timed 30 seconds and then double the figure to give the number of pulse beats per minute. The average adult rate is 72 beats per minute.

9 Keep your fingers on the pulse and continue so while you make the following additional observations:

(a) the regularity of the rhythm, which should be a pattern of evenly spaced beats;

(b) the volume of blood which dilates the artery at each beat: unless you have considerable experience in observing pulses you will find it difficult to say whether this is normal or not but perhaps you can form a general impression as to whether there is a full or a scanty volume of blood flowing along the artery;

(c) the tension of the artery wall: how easy is it to compress the pulse point so that the flow is interrupted and the beat stops?

10 When you have completed your observations, record them.

11 Ensure that the patient is left comfortable.

Chapter 6

Taking the oral temperature

The instrument used for taking the patient's temperature is a clinical thermometer. This usually has a scale from 35°C to 43°C. The normal body temperature (said to be 36.9°C or 37°C) is thus located reasonably within the scale.

1 Make sure that you have:

(a) a clinical thermometer in good order;

(b) a watch which displays seconds and minutes;

(c) some antiseptic swabs with which to wipe the thermometer after use.

2 Explain to the patient what you are going to do.

3 Check that within the last 15 minutes the patient has not had anything hot or cold to eat or drink.

4 Check the mercury level in the thermometer. If it is not already below 35°C, shake the thermometer until the mercury is down to below 35°C on the scale.

5 With the patient at rest, gently put the bulb end of the thermometer in his mouth and tell him to close his lips but not his teeth upon it. The aim is to keep it in place when you let go of it but not so that the patient bites it into two pieces while it is in position.

6 Tell the patient not to talk, cough, laugh, smile or sneeze. If any of these cataclysmic disturbances seems about to overcome him irresistibly, he must remove the thermometer before it is too late.

7 Leave the thermometer in place for two minutes.

8 Remove the thermometer gently, wipe it quickly clean with a swab and read the mercury level on the scale of the thermometer.
9 Record your reading.
10 Shake the thermometer down to below 35°C and restore it to its holder.
11 Ensure that the patient is comfortable.

Chapter 7

Counting the respiration

It is important that the rate of a patient's respiration should be counted without his being aware that it is being done. It is convenient to count the respiration after the pulse has been taken: so we suggest that if you have not already seen the section on taking the pulse you should turn to page 13 and read it now before going any further with the respiration.

1 Pretend that you are taking the pulse and hold the patient's wrist supported against his chest.

2 Count the rise and fall of the chest on inspiration and expiration: one rise plus one fall equals one respiration. Count the number that occur in one minute (60 seconds). The average normal adult rate is 16 to 20 respirations per minute.

3 Record your observations as to:

(a) rate;
(b) regularity;
(c) depth;
(d) absence or presence of sounds.

Chapter 8

Recording the blood pressure

1 Make sure that you have the necessary items of equipment. These are:

(a) a sphygmomanometer to measure the blood pressure;

(b) a stethoscope with which to listen to the arterial sounds of pulsation.

2 Explain to the patient what you are going to do.

3 The patient should be lying down comfortably and quietly at rest. You must help him to feel as relaxed as possible for tension in him can result in a reading which is falsely high.

4 Place the sphygmomanometer on a firm support close to the patient's arm which you propose to use for the measurement. Turn the apparatus so that he cannot see the scale.

5 Expose the patient's arm to well above the elbow by removing clothes or rolling up a sleeve.

6 Use your fingers to locate the pulsations of the patient's brachial artery. These are to be found above the elbow anteriorly at the medial margin of the biceps by pressure directed postero-laterally.

7 Wrap the cuff of the sphygmomanometer smoothly and firmly round the patient's arm, with the bag over the brachial artery and the tubes to the front. Tuck the end in to keep it securely in place.

8 Attach the tubing of the cuff to the manometer.

9 Using the stethoscope, apply its chest-piece to the patient's arm just below the band of the sphygmomanometer cuff and listen to the muffled sounds which are the pulsations of the brachial artery.

10 Continue to listen and use your other hand to inflate the cuff by using the bulb which is attached to it by tubing.

11 As you inflate the cuff, you will see the mercury rising up the scale of the manometer. Eventually a point is reached at which the sounds heard in the stethoscope have stopped because the brachial artery is fully compressed by the cuff.

12 Continue to listen while releasing the valve on the cuff so that the cuff slowly deflates and the mercury level slides down the scale.

13 A faint tapping sound heard in the stethoscope indicates that the pulse has re-established itself. Note the level of mercury at which this occurs. The level at which the sound is first heard is the systolic pressure.

14 Continue to listen and to deflate the cuff. The tapping becomes a loud knocking note as the systoles drive blood into the artery. As yet there is no sustained flow because of the compression from the cuff.

15 Suddenly the continuous flow is established and at that point the sound changes back to the muffled murmurous pulsations that you first heard before you inflated the cuff. Note the mercury level at that moment of change: this is the diastolic pressure.

16 Release all the air in the cuff, stop using the stethoscope and remove the cuff from the patient's arm.

17 Record the two levels of blood pressure.

18 Ensure that the patient is comfortable and put your equipment away tidily.

Chapter 9

Procedure for giving an enema

This set of instructions for giving an enema refers to an evacuant enema which is intended to stimulate the bowel to make it empty of faeces before a diagnostic X-ray examination. We are assuming that a disposable enema pack is used since this is now a widespread hospital practice. The disposable packs save time in preparing for, in carrying out and in clearing up after the procedure and they are so easy to use that a patient can self-administer an enema at home.

The enema pack consists of:

(a) a plastic bag or sac containing not more than 150 ml of a solution which is probably sodium phosphate or sodium acid phosphate;

(b) a short tube which is attached to the bag and enters it;

(c) a stoppered or guarded nozzle which is at the outer end of this tube.

Proceed as follows.

1 On a tray which is suitable for a clean (not sterile) procedure assemble the items you need. These are:

(a) the enema pack at room temperature;

(b) lubricating jelly and swabs or paper tissues;

(c) paper towels and a plastic sheet or an incontinence pad;

(d) a paper bag for discards;

(e) later, access to a lavatory or the use of a commode or

bedpan, lavatory paper and handwashing facilities for the patient.

2 Explain to the patient about the procedure and give him an opportunity to empty his bladder beforehand. Thereafter, the procedure will be more comfortable for him.

3 Ensure privacy for the patient.

4 Ask the patient to undress and put on a gown.

5 Take the patient to the place where the enema is to be given, assisting him as necessary, and ask him to lie down on the couch or bed on his left side. He should be lying with his buttocks close to the edge.

6 Place the paper towels and plastic sheet or the incontinence pad as protection for the bed under the patient.

7 Remove the stopper or guard from the nozzle of the rectal tube which is part of the enema pack.

8 Keeping the nozzle pointing upwards, lubricate it with a little lubricant on a swab or tissue.

9 Put your thumb over the inner end of the tube where it is inside the plastic sac. This manoeuvre stops the fluid from escaping when you turn the nozzle downwards as you must do for its insertion into the rectum.

10 Reassuring the patient, gently insert the nozzle and the tube into the rectum to an extent which is not more than 8–10 cm.

11 Release the compression of your thumb and squeeze or roll up the plastic sac so that all the solution is expelled into the rectum.

12 Withdraw the tube and discard the pack.

13 Encourage the patient to retain the enema for a few minutes, ensuring that he lies quietly and comfortably for this time.

14 With discretion, assist the patient as necessary for the evacuation of the enema. Do not leave him to manage it entirely alone.

Chapter 10

Laying up a sterile trolley

The general principles for laying up a sterile trolley apply consistently and do not vary with the purpose for which the trolley is being prepared. The same principles apply for the preparation of a tray for a sterile procedure. In this section we aim to set out the procedure for a trolley along general lines and leave the details of specific purposes to other pages in this book.

The two guiding rules which govern the procedure are:

(a) that you must preserve asepsis strictly;

(b) that you must use a 'no touch' technique.

1 Consider the area in which you are to prepare the trolley. It should be:

(a) spacious enough for the purpose;

(b) clean;

(c) well ventilated;

(d) away from people who may be talking, smoking, drinking coffee and generally relaxing;

(e) not part of a traffic route to other places and not part of a room where 'dirty' procedures are carried out (for example, dealing with bedpans and urinals);

(f) reasonably accessible and not remote from equipment which you need to prepare the trolley.

2 Ensure that the items which you need are assembled.

3 Wash and dry your hands (using a disposable paper towel or hot-air hand-drier).

4 Clean the lower shelf of the trolley and its uprights and supports using the preferred disinfectant. This can be applied with an aerosol spray or by means of paper towels used once only. Dry the surfaces with a paper towel.

5 Put on the lower shelf the items needed for the procedure about to be undertaken.

6 Immediately before the trolley is used, wash and dry your hands and clean the top of the trolley in the same way as for the rest of it. This newly cleaned top will serve to enclose the area of sterile activity. Some authorities consider that it need not be dry before use.

7 Use the top of the trolley as the working area from which to carry out the procedure which is to be undertaken for the patient, opening the sterile packs and handling the instruments by correct techniques which prevent the contamination of sterile areas and preserve asepsis.

8 After the procedure is complete, wash and dry your hands.

9 Clear the trolley, disposing appropriately of such items as instruments, dressings and lotions.

10 Clean the trolley again with disinfectant as before.

Chapter 11

Technique for a simple sterile dressing

This description is based upon the assumption that the dresser is an unassisted radiographer carrying out the procedure in the radiodiagnostic department.

1 Remember the basic principles that apply to the procedures of surgical dressing. These are:

(a) that wounds which are open and raw areas can become infected from the air;

(b) that the technique used should leave the wound exposed for a minimum length of time;

(c) that the wound may become infected from contaminated hands, instruments, lotions or other applications, dressings and by the droplet discharges of respiration;

(d) that strict attention must be paid to asepsis and to preserving the sterility of sterile areas and instruments and dressings.

2 Wash and dry your hands (disposable paper towel or hot-air dryer).

3 Prepare the tray or trolley for use (see page 22). The items you need to assemble for applying the dressing are:

(a) a sterile pack for a medium dressing;

(b) wound cleansing lotion if it is to be used (it may be provided already sterilized and ready for use in an individual plastic sachet);

(c) adhesive strapping to fix the dressing in place;
(d) a pair of scissors.

4 Remember to check the state of the sterile pack. It must be:
(a) intact;
(b) dry;
(c) clean-looking;
(d) not out of date;
(e) clearly labelled so that you know that you have the right one;
(f) showing evidence that it has been through a sterilizing procedure (for example, a printed statement or a striped tape).

If the pack fails to meet *all* these requirements replace it with one that does meet them.

5 When you open the sterile pack at stages **8** and **11** in this description, you should expect it to have the following contents (with some variations).

(a) An outer paper bag which is sealed. You can use this after it is empty to receive soiled dressings and other discards if you clip it fully open to the side of the trolley.

(b) An inner paper pack which is an enclosing paper towel to hold the other items which constitute the pack. You should find that this towel is folded in a special way with its corners turned out so that you can open it out by handling only the outside corners. This allows you to spread it on the trolley top and use it as a sterile working surface.

(c) Enclosed in the inner wrap are: (i) pairs of dissecting forceps; (ii) a plastic gallipot; (iii) swabs (cotton wool balls); (iv) dressings of gauze and wool.

6 Consider where you are to do the dressing, with regard to the appropriateness of the place (see page 22) and to the matter of privacy for the patient.

7 When you are ready, attend to the patient and explain what you are about to do. Make sure that the patient is comfortable.

You will be able to work more quickly and efficiently if you see to it that the patient is so positioned as to place horizontally the area to be dressed; then you will not have to fight the laws of gravity as you try to keep dressings in place.

8 When you have settled the patient, open the sterile pack's outer wrapping and shake the inner pack free on to the trolley top. Leave the inner pack unopened.

9 Prepare the patient by loosening strapping or bandages which may be keeping a previous dressing in place.

10 Wash and dry your hands as before.

11 Open the wrapping of the inner pack, using your fingers to touch only the edges, and spread it out over the trolley top, displaying the contents. This opened inner wrap is now the sterile area from which you work to do the dressing.

12 Use one pair of forceps in the pack to arrange the contents of the pack. You must handle these forceps very carefully, remembering that you must not contaminate any sterile items and that the handle of the forceps is unsterile once you have touched it. When you put down these handling forceps, place them in one corner of the sterile field nearest to you with their points directed inwards and the contaminated parts lying outside the sterile inner wrap.

13 Pour the lotion for the wound toilet into the sterile gallipot, remembering not to contaminate the gallipot or the lotion itself.

14 Use the handling forceps to remove any previous dressing and discard the forceps and the dressings. Disposable forceps and dressings both go into the 'discards' paper bag which you have clipped to the side of the trolley.

15 Take another pair of forceps from the sterile field and use them to pick up a swab, dip it into the lotion and clean the wound and its surroundings.

16 When swabbing the wound, observe the following points:

(a) use each swab for one sweep only and discard it into the paper bag as soon as it is raised from the skin surface;

(b) swab from the clean to the dirty end of the wound if you can see a difference;

(c) if the area is circular rather than linear, make each sweep one complete circle, beginning with an inner circular sweep and moving outwards.

17 In the same way as before, use dry cotton wool balls from the sterile field to dry the cleaned area.

18 Discard the forceps which you have used to swab and dry the wound.

19 Take another pair of sterile forceps and place gauze dressing over the wound to cover it completely.

20 Use strapping to fix the dressing securely and comfortably in place.

21 Ensure that you leave the patient in a settled, comfortable state.

22 Discard all the used materials into the paper bag which you are using for this purpose, close the top of the bag and place it on the trolley top.

23 Remove the trolley, discard the bag of used materials for incineration and take the trolley to where you prepared it.

24 Wash and dry your hands.

25 Clear and clean the trolley.

Chapter 12

Assisting with an intravenous injection

1 Ensure that you have assembled correctly, in the right place, all that is needed.

2 The requirements are as follows:

(a) the drug or agent for injection and a file for opening the ampoule which may contain it;

(b) a sterile syringe of appropriate size;

(c) a suitable sterile needle for the injection;

(d) a sterile filling-cannula;

(e) sterile swabs which today are often provided already impregnated with skin cleanser, each swab being individually packed in a sachet of metal foil which can be readily peeled open to allow the swab to be used;

(f) if necessary a suitable skin cleanser and a gallipot to hold it;

(g) a tourniquet or sphygmomanometer which may be used to distend and make prominent the vein which is selected for injection;

(h) a clean receiver;

(i) containers for discards as appropriate. Used swabs are likely to be put into a paper bag and needles and ampoules will go into a 'sharps' box.

3 Carefully check the drug or agent to be injected, paying attention to the following points:

(a) that it is the correct substance;

(b) that it appears to be in a suitable state and does not look unusual in regard to its colour, its translucency, its fluidity;

(c) that it is in a clearly labelled container which is not in any way damaged.

You must also make sure that the doctor who gives the injection checks what he is giving: you both share responsibility for this check.

4 Carefully identify the patient, reassuringly explain the procedure and see that the patient is comfortably settled where it is to be done.

5 Expose the injection site. This is usually one of the large superficial veins in front of the elbow.

6 Just before the procedure assemble the syringe. There are some possible variations here which are as follows.

(a) If there is only a small amount of the drug or agent to be injected, the needle to be used will attach directly to the syringe and may be used to serve both for drawing up the drug into the syringe and for injection subsequently into the chosen vein. In this case you proceed as follows. Snap open the case holding the sterile needle. Peel open the plastic wrap of the syringe and remove the syringe, holding it by the upper part of the barrel: do not touch the nozzle. Attach the needle (still in its case) to the syringe by inserting the nozzle of the syringe into the opening in the needle mount (you made this accessible when you took the top off the needle case). Put the assembled syringe and its still encased needle into the clean receiver to await use.

(b) If a large quantity of the agent is to be injected it is likely that the butterfly needle of an infusion set will be used for the injection and a wide-bore filling-cannula for drawing the agent into the syringe. In this case you proceed as follows. Open the upper end of the wrap of the cannula so that you have access to that end of the cannula which has an obvious mount for attaching it to the syringe. Peel open the plastic wrap of the syringe and remove the syringe, holding it by the upper part of the barrel: do not touch the nozzle. Join the syringe and the cannula by pushing the nozzle of the syringe into the opening in the cannula mount. Put the assembled syringe and the still wrapped cannula into the clean receiver to await use.

7 When the doctor is giving the injection, assist as required. Your tasks are likely to include the following:

(a) opening the ampoule or bottle;

(b) loading the syringe, with care for the preservation of the sterility of the inner parts and the nozzle of the syringe, the drawing-up cannula and the needles used;

(c) applying the tourniquet or inflating the sphygmomanometer cuff which you have applied to the patient's upper arm so as to constrict and distend the veins;

(d) supporting and holding steady the patient's arm;

(e) observing and reassuring the patient;

(f) cleansing the skin with sterile swab and skin cleanser;

(g) asking the patient to keep clenching and unclenching his fist to increase the distension of the veins in the arm.

(h) observing what the doctor is doing.

8 When the needle is in the vein and before the injection is given, you must release the constriction (tourniquet or sphygmomanometer cuff) on the arm. Watch carefully and you will see that the doctor checks that the needle has correctly entered the vein by slightly withdrawing the piston of the syringe. If blood immediately enters the syringe, then the needle is correctly placed and the injection can proceed. You may take this appearance of the blood as a signal to release the constriction: be careful not to dislodge the needle as you do it.

9 Afterwards, when the needle is withdrawn, you may be asked to apply a swab and firm pressure with your fingers to the injection site.

10 When convenient dispose of the used items appropriately, glass and needles going into the 'sharps' box.
11 Tidy away the other items.
12 Remain with and maintain observation of the patient.

Chapter 13

The use of oxygen

Oxygen may be given to patients when the normal supply of oxygen to their tissue-cells is not being maintained. Diagnostic radiographers are most likely to be closely involved with patients to whom extra oxygen is supplied in two contexts, as follows.

1 The patient is being given oxygen in an emergency situation in which he is in shock. His vital functions are depressed and the lack of fully-circulating blood is depriving his body-cells of oxygen. In these circumstances the oxygen is usually available in the department from a cylinder which contains it under pressure. It is given to the patient by means of a mask connected to the cylinder with tubing.

2 The patient is in a ward or in intensive care and for a time is being given continuous oxygen therapy. In this case the oxygen supply may be from a cylinder or from a piped supply to the bedside and it may be given to the patient in various ways:

(a) by mask;
(b) by intranasal tubes;
(c) in a plastic tent which encloses the bed and the patient;
(d) in an incubator if the patient is a neonate in a unit for the intensive care of babies.

Risks with oxygen therapy

Whatever your association with the use of oxygen, you must be fully aware of certain risks which arise. These are as follows.

1 Fire, since oxygen strongly supports combustion. The following precautions are to be observed:

(a) no smoking or naked lights;

(b) no electrical equipment operating when the oxygen supply is turned on and is in use;

(c) no oil, grease or spirit on the equipment or the patient, for oxygen is chemically reactive;

(d) remember the possibility of a spark from the discharge of static electricity produced from friction (the probability of such a spark is increased in the use of nylon clothing and bedding and in the combing and brushing of dry hair).

2 Risks to the patient's well-being from high concentrations of dry oxygen.

The radiographer's responsibilities

Below is a list of responsibilities for the radiographer which are related to the administration of oxygen.

1 Make sure that the cylinder which is to supply the patient is the correct black-and-white labelled cylinder.

2 Make sure that the cylinder is readily available in the department to bring to the patient without delay. It must be free from dust and be regularly checked for function. It should carry a label to show it as FULL, EMPTY, or IN USE.

3 Make sure that it is ready for use with a key or valve spanner and a pressure gauge attached to it.

4 Make sure that there are masks and appropriate tubing available for immediate use.

5 When you are attending a patient who is receiving oxygen you must observe the patient and the equipment which is being used. For the patient the important points are:

(a) colour;

(b) respiration;

(c) pulse;

(d) signals of distress (restlessness, anxiety, increased effort in breathing).

For the equipment, you must check:

(a) the flow rate of the oxygen;

(b) the tubing which carries the oxygen (for broken connections, kinks, obstructions);

(c) the mask (for faulty operation or incorrect placing so that it fails to cover the nose and mouth);

(d) that the supply is being maintained and has not ceased through the cylinder's becoming empty.

Chapter 14

Care before, during and after general anaesthesia

Before general anaesthesia

1 Be sure that oxygen, suction and the means for emergency resuscitation are available throughout the time that the patient is to be in the department.
2 Receive the patient with a greeting and reassurance.
3 Positively identify the patient, checking:
  (a) the identity bracelet worn;
  (b) his name as he gives it to you;
  (c) the patient's hospital number;
  (d) the patient's hospital notes;
  (e) the X-ray request form;
  (f) any previous radiographs.
4 Check that the patient is correctly prepared by considering these points:
  (a) suitable clothing;
  (b) the removal of dentures, spectacles, hearing aid;
  (c) jewellery or other items;
  (d) the premedication given;
  (e) the signed consent form.
5 Make the patient comfortable.
6 Do not leave the patient alone.
7 Keep yourself and others quiet.

8 If the patient speaks, reply quietly and appropriately.
9 Be ready to restrain the patient gently if he becomes restless and excitable.

During the induction and maintenance of general anaesthesia

1 Remain alert and observant.
2 Be ready to carry out instructions which may be given to you.
3 Remain quiet.
4 Do not leave the anaesthetist alone with the patient.
5 Remember that for a patient who is undergoing general anaesthesia the sense of hearing is the last one to leave and the first one to return. So be careful of what you say and the sounds that you make.

The termination of general anaesthesia

1 Remain alert and quiet.
2 Do not leave the patient alone.
3 Be ready to carry out instructions.
4 Observe the patient, checking for the following:
  (a) the colour of the skin and its state;
  (b) the respiration;
  (c) the pulse;
  (d) signs of haemorrhage, haematoma, oedema at the site of operation;
  (e) the level of consciousness.
5 Ensure that the patient has a maintained clear airway, keeping the inserted airway in place until he can remove it himself.
6 Remember that the semi-prone 'recovery' position is the safest for the patient if it is feasible.

7 If the patient is supine, hold his lower jaw forward.
8 As he recovers consciousness talk to him quietly and reassuringly.
9 Ensure the patient's comfort.
10 Arrange for the patient to be returned to the ward immediately after the instruction is given that he may leave the department.

Chapter 15

Accidents and dangerous occurrences

When an accident happens in your department certain procedures should be followed. These procedures fall within two separate categories:

(a) all the required undertakings for the first-aid care of the victim;

(b) all that is necessary for reporting and recording the accident.

First aid

The principles of first aid and particular techniques to be applied in some situations are topics considered in another part of this book so we do not need to expand them here. Care for the victim *must* be the immediate consideration even if little or no injury has been received. Simply on humanitarian grounds the questions 'Have you hurt yourself? Are you all right?' must be the first ones to which answers are sought.

Reporting and recording the incident

In the United Kingdom an Act of Parliament was passed which related to Health and Safety at Work. As a result, since 1981 there have been certain legal requirements with which health authorities and hospitals must comply in regard to accidents and dangerous occurrences which happen on their premises. These legal requirements involve recognized reporting and recording procedures which are to be followed whether or not anyone is injured: failure to follow these procedures constitutes a breach of the law.

We realize that not all who read this book are working in hospitals within the United Kingdom and are thus subject to these regulations. Nevertheless we felt that we would explain here some of their provisions. Other countries may have similar systems and even in the absence of laws and statutory instruments the stipulations here may give some guidelines for sound practice.

Within the statutory regulations of the United Kingdom, there are four main categories of incidents for which reporting and recording procedures have been stipulated. These are as follows.

1 *Dangerous occurrences.*

This is a term which embraces a number of clearly defined events such as the following: the collapse or overturning of a crane or hoist (for example in your department the ceiling-mounted tubestand comes down); bursting of a boiler; fire or explosion; collapse of a building; uncontrolled escape of dangerous agents; occupational exposure to pathogens which results in acute ill-health.

2 *Fatal accidents.*

These accidents are by definition those in which human life is lost.

3 *Major injury accidents.*

Major injuries are defined in the regulations and include fractures of the skull, the spine, the pelvis, arms and legs; amputations of limbs; loss of sight of an eye; other injuries which involve admission to hospital for longer than 24 hours.

4 *Other accidents.*

A special Report Form for Accidents and Dangerous Occurrences is in use and Table 1 displays for you the sequence of events for the reports and records which are required. We have interpreted the formalities of the published documents in terms of the X-ray department so that it is easier for inexperienced student radiographers to identify the people to which the stipulations refer. The

Table 1. Sequence of reports

1 Accident or dangerous occurrence happens.

↓

2 Report at once to the most senior person immediately available in the department (for example the radiographer with whom a student is working).

↓

3 Senior person investigates and immediately completes Part 1 of the Report Form.

↓

4 A doctor providing medical treatment completes Part 2 of the Report Form.

↓

5 The Head of the Department (Superintendent Radiographer) receives the Report Form, checks that it is properly completed so far, completes Part 3 of the Report Form and retains a copy.

↓

6 The Head of the Department sends the Report Form to the senior hospital administrator within 5 days.

7 At the time of the occurrence the local offices of the Health and Safety Executive organization must be told at once by telephone and in writing within 7 days if the events which have happened are dangerous occurrences, fatal accidents or major injuries accidents.

8 Hospital administrators must maintain a register of all these incidents and all accidents, the registers being annually reviewed.

most senior person who is immediately available may be a qualified radiographer who is supervising the student: in some circumstances such a radiographer will immediately report the incident to a more senior member of the department's staff.

Chapter 16

Actions in the event of a fire

1 At once raise the alarm by any or all of the following procedures:

(a) breaking the glass in a wall-alarm;

(b) dialling the emergency number and making a clear statement as to where the fire is;

(c) shouting.

2 Switch off any apparatus that is providing fuel for the fire, for example equipment powered by gas or electrical supply.

3 Move any people who are in immediate or impending danger.

4 Close doors and windows to reduce the air-supply to the fire and also to contain the smoke. Remember that smoke is extremely dangerous and that most people who lose their lives in a fire succumb to the toxicity of the smoke rather than to the heat of the flames.

5 If you have to try and combat smoke, remember two actions which may help you:

(a) covering your mouth and nose with a damp cloth such as a handkerchief, scarf or small towel which you have tied round your face;

(b) keeping low, for smoke tends to rise.

Instruct others in the same procedures.

6 If you can safely do so, remove whatever is obviously combustible and is near the fire. Examples are paper records, other burnable materials, cylinders of inflammable gases, inflammable chemicals.

7 If it is safe to do so, endeavour to control the fire by using the appropriate fire extinguishers or by smothering it with a fire blanket. Remember that you are better able to help your patients and your colleagues if you remain uninjured and alive and that your professional responsibility is to manage the situation and to look after others rather than to be hopelessly heroic. If you are fighting the fire, be careful to maintain a clear exit for yourself so that if it comes to the point where you must give in and retreat you can do so.

8 If someone's clothes catch fire, get the victim at once flat on the floor so that the smoke and flame and heat rise harmlessly (not up towards face and hair). Roll the person quickly and effectively in a covering such as a blanket to smother the fire.

9 Do not use any lifts. If the supply fails or is cut off they can become death-traps.

10 Once you have raised the alarm, avoid using the telephone. The lines may be very busy in the emergency.

11 Make sure that the fire-fighting team has all the help that you can give. Stay alert to clear exits and entrances, move people and carry out any instructions given to you by the fire-fighters.

12 If you have successfully fought and, you believe, extinguished a small fire remember that professional fire officers must be called to the scene to judge that it is now harmless and the situation is safe. It is better to feel slightly foolish in requesting the assessment of what may seem a relatively harmless incident than to be later appalled and surprised by the fire restarting.

Chapter 17

Radiological emergencies

A radiological emergency has occurred when a patient is endangered by an unfavourable reaction to the administration of a radiological contrast agent. Modern contrast agents exhibit much lower toxicity than those in early radiological use. Nevertheless minor adverse reactions sometimes occur; and on rare occasions the patient's malaise precipitates to a condition which is perilous to life, climaxing in cardiac and respiratory arrest.

Whilst these untoward events are improbable, experience shows that they are possible. They are most likely to happen when organic iodine compounds are introduced intravascularly in relatively large quantities during such investigations as intravenous urography and angiography. As a safeguard, radiographic rooms where these examinations are performed should include equipment for the rapid treatment of adverse reactions to radiological contrast agents.

Adverse reactions

Unfavourable reactions to contrast agents may be categorized as follows:

1 toxic effects of the injected chemical;

2 osmolar effects (the result of a shift of intracellular water through cellular membranes when these are subjected to assault by concentrated solutions);

3 allergic effects (an individual's idiosyncracy to a substance which is not toxic to the majority of people);
Some forewarning of the occurrence of **3** may be obtained if the patient is asked whether he knows he is allergic to any food or other substance, and whether he has a history of hay fever or asthma; in very few people is an allergy single. A radiologist or other doctor, before injecting a contrast agent, usually questions the patient about possible allergies.

Minor reactions to radiological contrast agents include:
1 transient sensations of warmth;
2 nausea and perhaps vomiting;
3 faintness and palpitations.

The following are actually or potentially much more serious and the radiographer must obtain immediate medical assistance for the patient who experiences any of these:
1 a skin rash (urticaria, which—even when it is mild—indicates allergy);
2 distressed breathing (bronchospasm);
3 difficulty in swallowing and breathing (laryngeal oedema);
4 collapse (analphylactic shock).

Emergency equipment

When radiological contrast agents are introduced to vessels and tissues during urography, arteriography and kindred procedures, equipment for the immediate treatment of a radiological emergency should be provided and always be present in the radiodiagnostic room. The items comprising this equipment may vary from hospital to hospital and readers of this book may wish to make their own inventories of what they find in their X-ray departments. Typically such equipment includes:
1 an alarm system;

2 an oxygen cylinder with a reducing valve and mask;
3 an airway for resuscitation;
4 a mouth gag;
5 a laryngoscope;
6 a sterile pack containing—
2x10 ml syringes
one 5 ml syringe
needles suitable for intravenous and hypodermic injection
2 fine exploring needles
a filling cannula
a pair of Mayo scissors
a large scalpel
a pair of dissecting forceps
2 pairs of Spencer Wells artery forceps
some gauze swabs;
7 a supply of drugs in suitable ampoules which may be used in resuscitation;
8 a suction apparatus;
9 a transfusion set;
10 a sphygmomanometer and stethoscope;
11 a tracheostomy set.

Chapter 18

Some first aid

The objectives of the techniques applied in first aid are:

1 to save life;
2 to prevent a worsening condition;
3 to promote recovery.

If you are acting to give first aid, your responsibilities are:

1 to assess the situation;
2 to identify the condition of the patient;
3 to give suitable first aid treatment at once;
4 to treat first the most urgent conditions;
5 to arrange if necessary for the patient to be properly transferred to medical or nursing care as appropriate.

The four most urgent serious conditions that require treatment are:

1 cardiac arrest;
2 respiratory arrest;
3 asphyxia;
4 haemorrhage.

} **all need action immediately.**

Cardiac arrest and respiratory arrest

Signs

1 Loss of consciousness.
2 No palpable arterial pulse (carotid artery in the neck).
3 Pallor and cyanosis.
4 Respiration and heartbeat have ceased.
5 Pupils become dilated after a minute or so.

Procedures for resuscitation

If the patient is unconscious and there is no carotid pulse, immediately begin a series of actions to achieve the following:
1 re-establishing the heartbeat by cardiac stimulation;
2 re-oxygenation of the lungs by pulmonary ventilation.
The actions to be taken are given below and the techniques to be used are shown in Table 2 and Table 3.
1 Place the patient supine on a firm surface.
2 Open his airway as follows:
(a) put one of your hands underneath the upper part of the patient's neck at the back;
(b) put your other hand on the patient's forehead and tilt his head back so that his chin juts vertically upwards;
(c) move your first hand from the back of his neck to the front and use it to push his chin upwards so that his tilted jaw will act to lift the tongue forwards and away from the oro-pharyngeal airway.
3 Clear the airway of any foreign matter in the patient's mouth by forming a hook-shape of the first two fingers of one of your hands and making a *quick* sweep round the inside of the mouth.
4 Maintain the patient's head in the open-airway position.
5 Carry out the procedures (see Table 2) for external chest compression and mouth-to-mouth ventilation in the following series.

Table 2. Procedures in resuscitation.

External chest compression	Checks for response	Mouth-to-mouth ventilation
1 With the patient supine on a firm surface, kneel beside the patient and thump the lower half of his sternum sharply with the ulnar border of your hand (this is precordial percussion). **2** Check for the heartbeat response. **3** If no response, place the heel of one of your hands on the centre of the lower half of the patient's sternum. **4** Cover this hand with your other one and lock the fingers of the two hands together, pressing on the sternum only and avoiding the ribs. **5** Keep your arms locked straight and rock forwards so that your arms are vertically above your hands and you are pressing down on the sternum using your body weight.	**1** Feel for the carotid pulse in the neck. If it is palpable, the heart is beating. **2** Look at the patient's face and lips for diminished cyanosis as a sign that oxygenated blood is circulating. **3** Bend over the patient and turn your head sideways to look along his chest and abdomen, your ear being close to his mouth. You will feel and hear his breath at your ear and will see the rise and fall of his chest.	**1** With the patient supine and his head tilted back to open the airway, maintain the position of his head with one of your hands, keeping your fingers beneath his chin and your thumb placed between his teeth to keep his mouth open. **2** Ensure that his face, mouth and neck are clear of obstructions and constrictions. **3** Clear his mouth with the fingers of your other hand. **4** Pinch the patient's nostrils closed by gripping them firmly between the bent middle and index fingers of your free hand. **5** Open your mouth wide and take in a deep breath. **6** Holding this breath, apply your own open mouth to the patient's mouth which you are

Continued

Table 2 – *continued*

External chest compression	Checks for response	Mouth-to-Mouth ventilation
6 Press the sternum downwards so that it moves about 3–5 cm (1–2 inches) towards the spine (this action compresses the heart between sternum and spine). **7** Rock back and slightly lift your hands to release the pressure. Steps **3** to **7** constitute one external chest compression.		holding open. Make sure that your lips form a close seal to his face and that his open mouth is entirely covered by your own. **7** Look along the patient's chest and blow your breath into his mouth, watching his chest rise as his lungs expand with the air you are breathing into them. **8** Lift your mouth clear of the patient's, watch his chest fall as the air goes out and take in another deep breath. **9** If the chest does not rise, check that the patient's head is in the right tilted-back position to open the airway and that the airway is clear. Steps **4** to **8** constitute one ventilation.

Table 3. Modifications to resuscitation procedures for infants and children.

External chest compression	Mouth-to-mouth ventilation
1 In a young child, compress at mid-sternal level (the heart is higher in the chest). **2** For neonates and infants, compress with two fingers only to move the sternum just 1.5–2.5 cm (0.5–1.0 inch). **3** In children between 5 and 10 years, compress with the heel of one hand only to move the sternum 2.5–3.5 cm (1.0 – 1.5 inches). **4** For older children, compress using both hands as for an adult but with lighter pressure. **5** Compress at a rate of 100 per minute (compare this with 80 per minute for an adult).	**1** Seal your mouth round both the nose and the mouth of the child. **2** Exhale your breath gently into the lungs. **3** Ventilate at a rate of 1 every 5 seconds (compare this with 1 every 4.5 seconds for an adult).

6 Make 15 external chest compressions. These should be done at a rate of 80 per minute, which means that you should do one compression every 0.75 second.
7 Check for the response of the heartbeat (see Table 2).
8 If no response, give two pulmonary ventilations (see Table 2).
9 Repeat the series of 15 compressions followed by two ventilations.
10 After 1 minute of this (let us say after you have done four of these compression-ventilation cycles) check for the heartbeat.
11 If there is no response, continue to repeat the cycle of 15 compressions followed by two ventilations.
12 Check for the heartbeat every 12 cycles (or every 3 minutes).
13 Continue until one of the following occurs:

(a) there is response and the patient's pulse and respiration are restored;

(b) someone qualified to do so takes your place in resuscitation;

(c) a doctor tells you to stop;

(d) you become physically exhausted and cannot effectively continue.

14 If the patient responds:

(a) stop the chest compressions immediately the heartbeat returns and the carotid pulse is found to be established;

(b) continue the mouth-to-mouth ventilation with one inflation every 4–5 seconds until the patient is breathing unaided;

(c) when the patient is successfully resuscitated with both the heartbeat and respiration restored place him in the semi-prone recovery position.

Asphyxia

Asphyxia is a condition in which the patient is not obtaining enough oxygen for the body-tissues. If unrelieved, it can quickly be fatal. There are many causes of asphyxia (as indicated in Table 4) and obviously the detailed procedures required of a trained first-aider are defined by the circumstances which have resulted in an asphyxiated patient. Since this book is not a manual solely of first aid, it has seemed best to give the student some signs and symptoms and some general procedures which form common factors in dealing immediately with asphyxia.

Signs

1 Obvious difficulty in breathing, the rate and the depth increasing.

Table 4. Asphyxia.

Conditions affecting airways and lungs	Conditions affecting respiratory control (brain centre/nerves)	Conditions affecting amount of oxygen present/used
1 Internal obstruction (a) tongue falling back (b) inhaled foreign body (c) oedema of the tissues **2** External obstruction (suffocation) **3** Presence of fluid in the airways **4** Compression of the airways/chest (a) strangulation and hanging (b) crush injury to the chest	**1** Electric shock injuries **2** Poisoning **3** Spinal cord injuries **4** Cerebral haemorrhage **5** Cerebral thrombosis	**1** Lack of oxygen available in the air, as in gas-filled and smoke-filled places **2** Change in atmospheric pressure **3** Carbon monoxide poisoning **4** Cyanide poisoning

2 Noisy respiration.
3 Cyanosis.
4 Possibly froth forming at the mouth.
5 Confusion and distress.
6 Possibly loss of consciousness.
7 Possibly respiratory arrest.

General immediate treatment

1 Seek to take the cause of the asphyxia from the patient or to remove the patient from the source of the asphyxia.

2 Ensure that the patient has an open airway (see page 48, steps **2**, **3** and **4**).

3 If the patient is not breathing begin artificial ventilation (see Table 2 on page 49) at once and give four inflations quickly.

4 Check the carotid pulse to discover if the heartbeat is present.

5 If the carotid pulse is present, repeat the mouth-to-mouth ventilations at a rate of one every 4–5 seconds until the patient can breathe naturally.

6 If the patient does not respond to the ventilations by re-establishing his own respiration, keep checking the carotid pulse after every four ventilations.

7 If the carotid pulse is not palpable proceed to the treatment for cardiac arrest and respiratory arrest.

8 When the patient is breathing unaided and has a palpable carotid pulse, place him in the semi-prone recovery position.

9 After resuscitation, continue to observe the patient and at 10 minute intervals check his pulse, his respiration and his level of consciousness.

10 Seek medical help as soon as you can.

Haemorrhage

The term haemorrhage means that there is a copious escape of blood from the blood vessels which normally contain it. The bleeding may be from a visible site and this is external haemorrhage: Table 5 shows three different types of bleeding which can be recognized as blood escapes from a wound. However, the bleeding may be at a place within the body, this being known as internal haemorrhage: internal haemorrhage may be indicated by the appearance of blood coming from a natural body orifice.

Table 5. Types of bleeding.

	Arterial	Venous	Capillary
Source	Damaged artery/ arteries	Damaged vein(s)	Damaged capillary vessels
Signs	Bright red colour (fully oxygenated) Ejected by spurts in rhythm with the heartbeat	Darker red colour (not oxygenated) Does not spurt but can gush copiously from a major vein	Colour is that of a mixture of arterial and venous blood Occurs in any wound, the blood oozing from the wound

Signs of marked blood loss

1 Evidence of a flow of blood.

2 Pallor.

3 Cold clammy skin.

4 Faster pulse rate but weaker pulse beat, which may become irregular.

5 Breathing shallow and rapid but the patient may sigh or yawn because of his need for more oxygen.

6 Patient is anxious and restless.

7 Patient feels weak, faint and giddy.

8 Patient may be thirsty.

9 Patient may be nauseated.

10 Patient may become unconscious.

Treatment for external haemorrhage

The aims are primarily to control the bleeding and secondarily to prevent a wound from becoming infected.

1 Major external bleeding is a serious emergency and requires immediate action to stop the bleeding, most especially if it is arterial bleeding.

2 Expose the wound.

3 Check for any visible foreign bodies and remove carefully any small superficial ones but do not spend much time on this. Large embedded foreign bodies may be better left since they may be serving usefully as plugs. You may worsen the situation as you pull them out.

4 Apply direct firm pressure to the bleeding wound with your fingers or the whole palm of your hand. If the wound is large, you may be able to draw and squeeze the edges together.

5 Lie the patient down, reassuring him.

6 If the wound is on a limb, elevate the limb unless you have reason to think that there might be fractures present.

7 Maintain the direct pressure with your hand until the blood-flow is visibly much reduced or has stopped.

8 Place a clean (preferably sterile) dressing over the wound to cover it completely and extend over its edges. Press it down and secure it firmly with a bandage so that pressure is maintained: remember that the bandage must not be so tight as to cut off circulation.

9 Treat the patient for shock (see page 58).

10 Seek medical aid.

11 In the case of arterial bleeding from a limb, if direct pressure on the wound cannot be applied or fails to arrest the haemorrhage then you can try indirect pressure. This is done by compressing a main artery at a point where it is close to bone. Table 6 shows the points at which to apply the pressure. Such pressure cuts off the supply to a limb so do not maintain it for longer than 15 minutes and regard it as a last resort.

Shock

Shock is a recognizable condition in which there is a general depression of physiological functions because the patient's body

Table 6. Points of pressure to arrest arterial haemorrhage.

The injured limb	Artery compressed	Point to apply manual pressure
The arm	The brachial artery	The inner side of the humerus about half-way between the medial epicondyle and the axilla. Press with your fingers firmly along the line that an inner sleeve-seam might follow. Press postero-laterally to flatten the artery against the bone.
The leg	The femoral artery	Press at a point on the front of the bony pelvis half-way between the symphysis pubis and the anterior superior iliac spine (it is about the midpoint of the groin-fold). Use your fist or the heel of your hand.

is without a full volume of circulating oxygenated blood. Shock can be caused by:

1 loss of blood from the vessels (haemorrhage);

2 loss of plasma (as would follow extensive burns);

3 loss of water (as would follow persistent vomiting and diarrhoea);

4 disturbance of the control of blood-circulation (as can follow the emotional experiences of great fear, horror, distress and pain).

Shock can be immediate or delayed. It can vary in degree from a state of weakness and faintness to a complete collapse even to the point of death.

Signs

1 Pallor.
2 Cold clammy skin.
3 Faster pulse rate but weaker beat of the pulse, which may become irregular.
4 Shallow breathing at an increased rate and the patient may sigh and yawn as he seeks to take in more oxygen.
5 Patient is anxious and restless.
6 Patient feels weak, faint and giddy.
7 Patient may be nauseated.
8 Patient may be thirsty.
9 Patient may become unconscious.

Procedures in first aid

1 Reassure the patient.
2 If the patient is conscious, is not vomiting and is having no difficulty in breathing then position him (if you can and his state allows it) lying supine at rest with his head turned to one side.
3 Preferably his heels should be positioned slightly higher than his head. This is easy if the patient is on a tilting X-ray table. If he is not so fortunately placed, raise his legs on pillows or rolled-up blankets (unless there may be or are certainly fractures).
4 If the patient vomits, appears to have difficulty breathing, shows a falling level of consciousness or becomes unconscious, then he should be placed in the semi-prone position of recovery unless he has injuries which preclude this. If you cannot move him from the supine position, then you must maintain a clear

airway for him by holding his head tilted back with the jaw held forwards and upwards.

5 If the patient's condition deteriorates to cardiac and respiratory arrest, at once begin resuscitation (see page 48) and send for help.

6 Keep the patient warm by covering him with a blanket.

7 Do not use any positive applications of heat such as hot-water bottles since these result in an increased blood-flow to the skin with deprivation of vital structures.

8 Loosen any of the patient's clothing which is tight.

9 If the patient is thirsty, you may moisten his lips with water but do not let him have anything to drink.

10 If you have a shocked patient in your care in the X-ray department while he is being examined you must remember the following rules of guidance:

(a) reassure him;

(b) keep him lying down;

(c) keep him warm and conserve his energy;

(d) keep him under observation for changes in pulse, respiration, colour and level of consciousness;

(e) keep to the necessary minimum the length of time that he must spend in your department and ensure that the radiographic procedures are carried out efficiently and quickly.

Loss of consciousness

Consciousness is defined as the responsiveness of the mind to the impressions received through the senses: anyone who becomes completely unconscious is not receiving sense impressions and there is no response in the mind. Loss of consciousness results from interference in the functioning of the brain and there are many possible causes. We think that it is important for radiographers to observe patients knowledgeably and to recognize different levels of consciousness so that they may assess deterioration or improvement in a patient's condition. Table 7 sets out the important facts.

Causes of unconsciousness

If a patient becomes unconscious while he is in your care or you are called to give aid to a patient who has become unconscious, it is important that you try to decide the cause of the unconsciousness and thus identify the situation with which you are dealing. You need answers to the following questions.

1 What was the onset? Gradual or sudden? Silent or accompanied by any crying out? Preceded by any accident or incident or known condition which explains it? Is there visible injury?

2 What is the level of consciousness?

3 Is the patient pale? Flushed? Cyanosed?

4 Is the skin dry? Moist? Hot? Cold?

5 Is the pulse-beat present? Slow? Fast? Weak? Strong? Regular? Irregular?

Table 7. Levels of consciousness.

State	Patient's level of activity
Fully conscious	Aware of surroundings Replies to questions Engages in conversation
Drowsy	Will answer direct questions Answers vaguely when addressed Can obey commands
Stuporous	Responds to painful stimuli
Comatose	Completely unconscious and without response to pain.

(Arrows beside table: ↑ Improving; ↓ Deteriorating)

6 Are the patient's respirations normal? Regular or irregular? Is the rate fast or slow? Is breathing silent or noisy? Is there any smell on his breath?
7 Are the limbs and body slack? Rigid? In spasmodic muscular contraction?
8 Is there incontinence of urine or faeces?
We give below some points in the general care of an unconscious patient and some first aid procedures for certain states which produce a loss of consciousness.

General care of an unconscious patient

1 Do not leave the patient alone.
2 See that the patient has a maintained clear airway by:
(a) if necessary, making sure that his mouth is clear of obstructions such as displaced teeth, false teeth, vomit, blood;
(b) maintaining him in the semi-prone recovery position;
(c) holding his head tilted back with the jaw forwards and upwards, if he must lie supine.
3 Observe the patient and check for:
(a) colour and state of skin;
(b) cyanosis;
(c) pulse;
(d) respiration;
(e) level of consciousness.
4 Be alert for signs of change and begin resuscitation if the patient has cardiac/respiratory arrest.
5 If the patient recovers consciousness, reassure and help him and maintain observation while he is in your care.

Loss of consciousness in diabetes mellitus

Diabetes mellitus is a disorder which results in a deficiency of the secretion of the hormone insulin by the pancreas. Insulin functions to control the metabolism of sugar. If the supply of insulin fails the level of sugar in the blood rises (this is hyperglycaemia) and if this state is prolonged the patient will become unconscious and eventually will die.

Diabetes mellitus is not a curable disease but it can be controlled by treatment and the blood sugar can be stabilized to keep a normal level. This control is achieved by:

1 maintaining the patient on a diet which is correctly balanced in regard to carbohydrate, fat and calorific values;

2 administering measured amounts of insulin.

If the patient receives too much insulin relative to the amount of sugar which he takes, his blood sugar falls to an abnormally low level (this is hypoglycaemia). If this state is uncorrected the patient rapidly becomes unconscious and eventually will die.

There are thus two forms of unconsciousness associated with diabetes mellitus: one linked to hyperglycaemia (raised blood sugar) and one linked to hypoglycaemia (low blood sugar). Table 8 sets out the important facts that you should know. Below we give the first aid treatment for a diabetic patient who becomes suddenly faint and unconscious in your department: hypoglycaemia is most likely to be the cause of this.

Treatment for hypoglycaemia

1 If the patient is not yet unconscious and can swallow, you must at once give him something sugary by mouth: sugar itself, a sweetened drink, chocolate, sweet biscuits, sweet fruit juice. Ask him if he has any sweets or sugar with him.

2 Support him and reassure him.

3 If the patient becomes unconscious proceed to the general

Table 8. Loss of consciousness in diabetes mellitus.

State	Blood sugar level	Signs	Needs
Diabetic coma Slow onset. The cause is lack of insulin.	Hyperglycaemia (high blood sugar)	Drowsiness. Eventual unconsciousness. Deep stertorous breathing. Breath smells of acetone. Skin is dry.	Insulin
Insulin coma The onset can be rapid with early warning signs not apparent, especially in a patient who has been receiving insulin treatment for many years. The cause is too much insulin relative to the intake of carbohydrate.	Hypoglycaemia (low blood sugar)	Sinking feeling and hunger. Faintness. Eventual loss of consciousness. Quiet shallow breathing. No smell of acetone on the breath. Moist clammy skin.	Glucose

care of the unconscious patient and seek medical aid at once since a doctor will be needed quickly to give glucose intravenously.

4 If the patient does not lose consciousness, seek medical advice before he leaves your care.

Loss of consciousness: epileptic attacks

Epilepsy is a disease in which there are brief disturbances in the normal electrical impulses activating the brain. When these disturbances occur, the patient undergoes an epileptic attack (epileptic fit, epileptic seizure). Epilepsy has been categorized in regard to two degrees of severity of the attacks which occur:
1 major epilepsy in which the patient loses consciousness during the attack;
2 minor epilepsy in which the patient has impaired awareness during the attack but does not lose consciousness.
Table 9 sets out some facts.

First aid in major epileptic attacks

1 If you can catch the patient as he falls, try to break the fall and ease him gently to the ground.
2 If the patient is already on the ground or is lying on an X-ray table, examination couch, bed or stretcher, leave him as he is unless it is imperative that he be moved from some dangerous situation.
3 If you can, loosen clothing round the patient's neck and place something soft under his head.
4 When the convulsions begin remember that your part must be relatively inactive. You must aim to protect the patient from injury if you can.
5 Observe the following prohibitions:
- (a) do not forcibly restrain the convulsive movements;
- (b) do not move the patient unless the situation is dangerous;
- (c) do not put anything into the patient's mouth;
- (d) do not try to prise open the patient's mouth;
- (e) do not try to rouse the patient from his unconscious state.

Table 9. Epilepsy.

The condition	Signs during the attack	
Major epilepsy Stage 1 is very brief Stage 2 lasts a few seconds Stage 3 lasts 1 minute or so Stage 4 lasts up to about 5 minutes Stage 5 lasts for several minutes up to 1 hour	Stage 1	Patient may be aware of a warning sensory disturbance (an aura) which tells him he is going to have an attack
	Stage 2	(a) Sudden loss of consciousness, sometimes with an outcry (b) Rigidity (c) Cyanosis (d) Absence of breathing (e) Eyes turned upwards
	Stage 3	(a) Muscles relax (b) Convulsions (contraction and relaxation of groups of muscles) occur (c) Vigorous uncontrolled movements of limbs and body (d) Foam, possibly bloodstained, round the mouth (e) Noisy difficult breathing through a clenched mouth (f) Possibly incontinence of urine/ faeces
	Stage 4	(a) Muscles relax and convulsions cease (b) Patient remains unconscious
	Stage 5	(a) Return to consciousness (b) Patient feels dazed and confused (c) Patient may act strangely (d) Patient wants to remain at rest
Minor epilepsy	(a) Appearance of daydreaming (b) Unfocused eyes staring ahead (c) Possibly strange behaviour and speech (d) Possibly loss of memory	

6 When the convulsions have ceased, turn the unconscious patient into the semi-prone recovery position.
7 Stay with the patient until you are sure that he has regained full consciousness.
8 Seek medical advice as to what should be done for the recovered patient.
9 Do not send the patient home alone.

First aid in minor epileptic attacks

1 Remain inactive, aiming only to:
- (a) protect the patient;
- (b) keep other people away from the patient;
- (c) talk to the patient reassuringly and quietly.

2 Stay with the patient until you are sure that he has recovered his full normal consciousness.
3 Be alert to the possibility that a major epileptic attack might soon follow the minor episode.
4 Report the occurrence and seek medical advice as to what should further be done for the recovered patient.

Loss of consciousness: fainting attack

A simple fainting attack is a transient loss of consciousness caused by a temporarily impaired blood supply to the brain.
Possible causes are:
1 emotional;
2 nervous reaction to pain;
3 exhaustion;
4 lack of food;
5 lack of fresh air;
6 a long period of physical inactivity in an erect posture.

Signs

1 Pallor.
2 Visible facial sweating.
3 Pulse is slow and weak.
4 Patient feels weak and giddy.
5 Patient may feel nauseated.
6 Patient may feel thirsty.
7 Patient may breathe rapidly, may yawn or may sigh.
8 If the patient passes into unconsciousness, recovery is quick and is complete in only a minute or two.

First aid procedures

1 Immediately seek to forestall the state of unconsciousness by restoring the blood flow to the brain. Do this either:

(a) by seating the patient and leaning him well forward and down with his head hanging low between his knees:

OR

(b) by lying the patient flat, preferably with his head lower than his heels.

2 Tell the patient to take deep breaths.
3 Reassure the patient.
4 If the patient is unconscious, treat as for general care of the unconscious patient.
5 Loosen tight clothing.
6 Ensure a plentiful supply of fresh air.
7 As he recovers, maintain reassurance for the patient and help him to become upright again.
8 When you are sure that the patient is recovered and is fully conscious, you may give him water to sip if he says that he is thirsty.
9 If you are worried about the patient or he seems very slow to recover, seek medical advice.

Injuries from electricity

When a person is injured by electricity he is said to have received an electric shock: this term means that the person has had an electric current passing through his body from an external source. The results of this are variable with the circumstances in which the accident occurs and so the first aid procedures to be applied are also varied to meet the conditions to be found in the victim of the electricity. The conditions which may result from an electric shock are:

1 cardiac arrest;
2 respiratory arrest;
3 burns;
4 fractures;
5 shock.

What the first aider must do is to treat as many of these conditions as may be found, following the basic principles which aim to save life and to treat first the most urgent life-threatening conditions.

In the case of the victims of electric shock, the first thing to be done is to break the contact between the patient and the source of the electric current. You must remember that you do this while keeping yourself isolated from the electricity. If you fail to isolate yourself you may easily fail in your rescue of the patient and there will be two people (the patient and yourself) in need of first aid help from a third.

With the foregoing in mind, we set out below some general instructions for first aid help in the case of an accident with electricity in your department.

1 Break the contact between the victim and the electrical source. Consider the following:

(a) switching off at the mains supply switch;
(b) pulling a plug from a wall socket;
(c) pushing or pulling the patient away from the source.

If you cannot switch off and must try to remove the patient from the live source, remember the following:

(a) you can insulate yourself by standing on a dry insulating surface (wood, rubber matting, folded newspapers);

(b) you should use an insulating material (wooden pole, broomstick, a length of rope) to push or pull the patient away from the live source;

(c) you must not use anything metallic;

(d) you must not touch the patient's skin with your bare hands;

(e) you must avoid dampness.

2 With the patient and yourself safe from further electrical injury, quickly assess the state of the patient and identify the conditions to be treated.

3 Proceed immediately with the required first aid, treating first the most serious and urgent condition.

4 Refer the patient for medical attention as soon as you can even if the injury appears to you to have been slight.

Fractures

In medical terminology a fracture is a broken bone. Fractures may be categorized according to type and in Table 10 the varieties are listed and explained.

Signs

1 Pain or tenderness at the site of the injury.

2 Possibly obvious deformity at the fracture site.

3 Loss of function such that the patient may not be able to move the involved part easily or indeed at all.

4 The patient may have heard or have felt the snap of breaking bone.

Table 10. Fractures.

Type	Definition
Closed fracture (Simple fracture)	A fracture in which the skin is not broken, there is no open wound communicating with the fracture site, there are no complications.
Compound fracture (Open fracture)	The skin is broken and there is an open wound leading down to the fracture site. There may or may not be a broken bone protruding through the wound.
Complicated fracture	In addition to the broken bone there is an associated injury in which the broken bone has damaged a nerve or an important adjacent organ; or when the fracture is associated with a dislocated joint.
Comminuted fracture	A fracture in which the bone is fragmented, splintered, crushed into several small pieces.
Greenstick fracture	A fracture in which one edge of a bone is broken and the opposing edge is simply bent. This is common in children.

5 Swelling of the injured part. The breaking bone is bound to damage blood vessels and a varying amount of blood escapes into the tissues. In some cases (for example a fractured femur) the loss of blood can be as great as 20–30 per cent of the whole volume. So a later sign is bruising as this extravasated blood reveals itself.

6 A sign that a doctor attending the patient may seek is the coarse bony grating noise (crepitus) as the broken ends move against each other. This may be felt or heard as the injured part is examined. You should not seek the sign yourself but you may inadvertently elicit it and when you do detect the crepitus then you know at once that there is a fracture present.

General principles in first aid for fractures

1 If there is doubt, you must treat the patient as if it were certain that there is a fracture present.
2 Treat first the most serious condition present: cardiac arrest, respiratory arrest, severe haemorrhage and difficulty in breathing all take precedence over fractures.
3 Ensure that there is no aggravation of the injury by movement at the fracture site. To this end observe the following points:

- (a) do not move the injured part unnecessarily;
- (b) as appropriate, steady and support the injured part by hand; by the use of firm padding placed against the part; by the application of a sling; by securing the injured part to a sound part with padding and firm bandages; by the use of a splint.

4 If it is necessary to lift the patient you must make sure that there are enough people to do the lifting and that special attention is given to supporting and steadying the injured part.
5 Treat for shock.

Burns and scalds

Burns and scalds are both injuries from contact with heat, the burn originating from dry heat and the scald from moist heat. In giving immediate treatment, you must be guided by the following imperatives.
1 Reduce the heat and its effects.
2 Prevent infection.
3 Minimize shock.
4 If the burning is extensive transfer the patient urgently to medical care.

General guidelines for first aid for burns

1 Cool the burned part by covering it with a slow flow of cold water from a running tap or by immersing it in a bowl of cold water. Maintain this until the pain and heat have diminished (10 minutes or longer).
2 Cover the burned area with a dressing that is clean (best if it is sterile), is not fluffy or rough and is not adhesive.
3 Do not interfere with the burned area by such activities as breaking blisters, pulling off loose clothing or charred skin, applying lotions, fats or ointments.
4 Reassure the patient and watch for signs of shock.
5 If you are in any doubt about the patient, seek medical help.

Minor wounds involving broken glass

If someone is wounded in an incident which involves broken or shattered glass, you must decide whether or not there are fragments of glass within the wound and you must be careful to avoid further embedding of any foreign bodies by the treatment you give.
1 Look carefully for any visible glass fragments that are superficial and are easily picked off. If you see them, remove them carefully, preferably using sterile forceps. If there is a large fragment of glass obviously deeply embedded, it is better to leave it alone since you may make the injury worse as you pull it out.
2 Control the bleeding by pulling the edges of the wound together and holding them firmly in contact with each other. As you do this, try to avoid pressure on any embedded piece of glass which you can see sticking out.
3 Apply a dressing to the wound in such a way as to avoid pressure on a protruding embedded glass fragment. To this end you can consider the following possibilities:

(a) a gauze dressing may have a hole cut in it to pass over the embedded fragment;
(b) pieces of gauze may be placed alongside and around the fragment;
(c) pads of cotton wool may be made ring-shaped and built up around the glass fragment so as to be high enough to shield the glass from pressure which would drive it inwards;
(d) a firm bandage can be applied to cover the dressings in such a way that it does not at all cover the protruding glass. You can wind on the bandage in a diagonal or a figure-of-eight arrangement formed to skirt the protruding glass.

4 Seek medical advice about the patient with reference to further exploration and treatment of the wound and the removal of any glass fragments.

Chapter 19

An infectious patient in the ward

An infectious patient who is being barrier nursed in the ward is in a single room.

Outside the room should be the following:

1 the patient's notes;

2 a supply of disposable masks of the filter type;

3 a pedal bin for discarded masks;

4 a plastic bag in a colour coded for the disposal of contaminated materials to be burnt;

5 facilities for hand-washing with a supply of paper towels.

Inside the room should be the following:

1 two gowns, each on its separate coathanger, available just inside the door;

2 a supply of items needed for nursing (examples of these are washing equipment, linen, plastic covers and bags, paper towels, disposable bedpans and urinals, a commode);

3 a plastic bag colour coded for the disposal of contaminated linen;

4 the patient, of course!

Procedure for the radiographers

1 Prepare all the equipment that you plan to take, cleaning it with a disposable cloth moistened with disinfectant or by the light use of a disinfectant aerosol spray.

2 Make sure that you have disposable covers for cassettes which are to be in contact with the patient.
3 With the equipment, go to the ward and announce yourself, establishing that you may now X-ray the patient.
4 Outside the patient's room, wash your hands and put on a mask.
5 Go into the room with the equipment, closing the door after your entry.
6 Greet the patient and explain the procedure.
7 Remember that the outsides of the gowns are considered to be contaminated and that the insides are considered to be clean and free from contamination.
8 Each radiographer should put on a gown, taking care not to touch the outside or to contaminate the inside of the gown by touching it with any of the outer surfaces.
9 Undertake the radiography as required. It is best if one radiographer handles only the equipment and not the patient, while another handles only the patient and not the equipment.
10 When the radiographic examination is complete and the patient is tidy and comfortable, wash your hands and dry them on a paper towel in the room.
11 Take your leave of the patient.
12 Take off the gown and restore it to its coathanger, taking care not to touch the outside of it or to contaminate the inside from the outside.
13 With the equipment leave the room, closing the door behind you.
14 Discard the mask, touching only the tapes.
15 Clean the equipment as before.
16 Wash and dry your hands outside the room before you leave the ward.

Chapter 20

An infectious patient in the X-ray department

1 Make sure that the patient comes at a time when the department is not busy.
2 Make sure that all is ready in the X-ray room and that the patient immediately on his arrival in the department may be brought to the room where he is to be examined.
3 Remember that the patient should remain in this room throughout the time that he is in the department, including any periods of waiting.
4 Two radiographers should reserve themselves for this patient while he is in the department.
5 Disposable covers must be used for any cassettes which are to be in contact with the patient.
6 The radiographers should wash their hands and put on gowns and masks.
7 Greet the patient, identify him and explain the procedure.
8 Undertake the radiographic examination as required. One radiographer should handle only the equipment and not touch the patient. The other radiographer should handle the patient and not touch the equipment, except for the X-ray table/erect bucky/film-holder as may be necessary while positioning the patient.
9 The radiographer who has not handled the patient should be

the one to leave the room to take cassettes to the film-processor or to check the processed radiographs.

10 If they have been in contact with the patient, cassettes should be wiped with disinfectant before they leave the room. This job should be done by the radiographer who has not been handling the patient.

11 When the patient is ready to leave the department, you must ensure that he returns to the ward without delay, remembering that he must remain in the X-ray room until he goes. Remember to say goodbye to the patient.

12 After the patient has left, wash and dry your hands.

13 Remove gowns and masks, disposing of them appropriately.

14 Clean all the equipment with disinfectant.

15 Wash and dry your hands before proceeding to anything else.

Chapter 21

The patient with a tracheostomy

Tracheostomy is a surgically made opening into the trachea for the purposes of maintaining an airway against obstruction of the larynx; of assisting ventilation in the pulmonary management of patients who are unconscious or paralysed or suffering from a chest disease; of aspirating secretions from the trachea and bronchi. The tracheostomy may be temporary (and most are) or it may be permanent.

A tracheostomy tube is a wide-bore tube which is especially shaped in a curve for insertion in the surgically made opening and down the trachea. It is used to keep the opening patent and allow access to the trachea for as long as the tracheostomy is to be maintained. A tracheostomy tube may be plastic or metal and it has attached to it tapes which fasten around the patient's neck and hold the tube in place.

Radiographers will not be concerned with the sustained and meticulous nursing care which is so important following a tracheostomy but they will certainly encounter patients with tracheostomies, be they temporary or permanent. Here we outline some important points for the care which the radiographer must provide.

1 Reassure the patient always and be ready to interpret his endeavours to communicate with you. He needs help here because he cannot use his voice unless the tracheostomy is long-standing and he has been given training in speech-production. So provide pencil and paper and wait patiently for *all* that he is trying to convey.

2 Observe the patient alertly. Look for any attempts to communicate and for signs of inadequate airway and ventilation: that is, for cyanosis and visible respiratory distress.

3 Observe the tube to see that it maintains itself securely in the right place. A tube which is partially or totally displaced is very dangerous and must be adjusted as soon as possible.

4 Observe the tapes to ensure that they remain secure and are neither too tight nor too loose.

5 Unless the tracheostomy is long-standing the patient must remain attended and must not be left alone.

6 Suction apparatus should be available as long as the patient is in the department.

Chapter 22

Tracheo-bronchial suction

It may be necessary to use suction apparatus on a patient in order to clear the airways of mucous secretions. Patients who cannot clear their own airways by effective coughing are, of course, at the risk of asphyxiation and it is to such patients (who may or may not have undergone tracheostomy) that suction apparatus (often called a sucker) may be applied. In an emergency you must be ready to act quickly and bring the apparatus into operation without wasting time.

The sucker uses vacuum suction at a pressure of 100–120 mm of mercury. The apparatus may be:

1 electrical and so requiring connection to a mains outlet by the usual arrangement of a lead-cable and a plug to fit the socket from which it is to be powered;

2 independent of a mains supply, being operated by a foot-pump;

3 a fixed installation, the unit and its controls being wall-mounted.

In the X-ray department the electrical sucker mounted on a castered trolley is the type most likely to be encountered.

Tracheo-bronchial suction by means of apparatus is a sterile procedure which must be carefully undertaken. The items required are as follows.

1 The suction apparatus in full working order, including the plug used to connect it to the mains socket outlet if the equipment is of that type.

2 A trolley or tray for other equipment. This must be prepared as for any sterile procedure: see page 22.

3 Sterile disposable suction catheters. Each catheter is pre-sterilized and is in its own separate paper pack. The catheters are in various sizes and have at least one side-opening as well as an open end (described as whistle-tipped catheters). The size 14FG is appropriate for most adults: if there is a tracheostomy tube in place the selected size of catheter should be half the diameter of the tracheostomy tube.

4 Sterile suction tubing and connector which will provide the means to attach the catheter to the sucker.

5 Sterile disposable gloves.

6 Some suitable sterile lubricant for the catheter and the means to apply it to the catheter tip: for example a sterile gallipot to hold the lubricant, into which the tip of the catheter may then be dipped.

7 Clean water in a clean bowl.

8 A large disposable bag which can be conveniently clipped to the handle of the sucker.

The procedure is as follows.

1 If the patient is conscious, explain the procedure simply and reassuringly.

2 Prepare the trolley-top or tray as for a sterile procedure and lay out on it the items which you need, as listed above.

3 Check that the sucker is in good order, is near the patient and is conveniently connected to a socket outlet if that is required.

4 Ensure that the patient is placed in a position that gives easy access to the tracheostomy tube if you are to suck through that or to his mouth if no tracheostomy has been done: a suitable posture is the supine one with neck extended.

5 Wash your hands, unless the situation is very urgent.

6 Open the connection-end of a catheter pack: this is recognizable by the coloured plastic mounting-piece on the end of the catheter. With your fingers, draw this end clear of its wrapping leaving most of the rest of the catheter still enclosed.

7 Attach the catheter to the suction apparatus through the connector and tubing.

8 Put a sterile glove on your dominant hand and remove the catheter from its pack, being very careful lest the catheter become contaminated through contact with anything unsterile as you withdraw it and hold it in your gloved hand.

9 With your ungloved hand turn on the suction.

10 Use your ungloved hand to close the catheter to suction by folding it in a bend against the connection point.

11 Lubricate the catheter tip, dipping it into the gallipot which holds the lubricant.

12 If there is a tracheostomy tube in place, gently introduce the catheter into the tube and push it down as far as it will easily go: this is to the level where the trachea bifurcates and there is a ridge which separates the openings of the right main bronchus and the left main bronchus. If there is no tracheostomy tube, put the catheter gently into the patient's open mouth and pass it over the back of the tongue as far as he finds it tolerably acceptable.

13 Release the folded catheter in your ungloved hand so that suction is applied and then begin slowly to withdraw the catheter by a rotating action: the catheter is of course sucking as it goes. Once the catheter is withdrawn it must not be used again and so a new one and a new sterile glove must be taken if it is decided to make a second application. While the catheter is in the trachea, the patient may find it difficult to breathe so you should consider applying the suction for only so long a period as you can easily hold your breath (assuming that you have normal ability here and have not had special practice in under-water swimming or singing!).

14 When you have finished with them discard the glove and catheter into the disposable bag.

15 Remember to observe your patient throughout, watching especially for cyanosis and signs of respiratory distress.

16 Clean the suction tubing and connector by sucking water through it from the bowl which you have ready.
17 Turn off the suction equipment.
18 Wash your hands.

Chapter 23

The patient with a colostomy/ileostomy

Colostomy is a surgical operation which brings some part of the colon to an opening on the surface of the abdomen. Through this opening the faeces are discharged: they are not passed from the rectum at the anus, which is the normal and controllable outlet. A colostomy may be temporary or it may be permanent.

Ileostomy is a surgical operation which brings the ileum to an opening on the surface of the abdomen. Faecal material drains to the outside through the passage surgically made: it no longer is conveyed through to the colon for controlled discharge from the rectum in the normal way. Ileostomy is usually permanent.

In both these operations an artificial opening is made between an internal passage (the colon or the ileum) and the body's surface (the anterior abdominal wall): such a surgically made opening is called a stoma (the plural word is stomata). Radiographers should recognize some features in the special care of patients who have undergone colostomy or ileostomy and we give below a few points of importance.

1 You need to remember that this patient no longer has voluntary control over the discharge of faecal matter. This makes him feel at a great disadvantage socially. Because we tend to have a sense of shame and humiliation when there is such loss of control, we are reluctant to reveal the situation and we seek concealment. So the radiographer's attitude must be one in which consideration, understanding and reassurance are carefully

blended with a matter-of-fact acceptance of the difficulties. The radiographer must give competent assistance in the practical situation and must display no uncertainty, apprehension or disgust.

2 In modern practice a disposable, plastic stoma bag is used to contain the faecal matter which discharges itself through the stoma. The bag is kept in contact with the wall of the abdomen by a self-adhesive plaque. A hole in the centre of the plaque fits round the stoma and the opening of the bag fits firmly to the plaque by means of a flange which guards the opening. The arrangement is intended to ensure that the faecal matter when it ejects through the stoma is caught and held in the bag. The bag may be drainable through its lower end and emptied as often as necessary, being replaced with a new one every 3 days. Or it may be removed when it is full by detaching it from the flange. It is then discarded and replaced with a new one.

3 An important consideration is the state of the skin round the stoma. Unless care is taken, the skin can become painfully and depressingly excoriated by the enzymes in the intestinal fluid. So the skin must be kept clean and protected.

4 To help these patients, you may be required to implement any or all of the following:

(a) provision of new stoma bags;

(b) provision of privacy and the use of a lavatory;

(c) provision of washing facilities;

(d) assistance as required with emptying stoma bags, renewing stoma bags, washing the stoma;

(e) catheterizing the bowel through the stoma in giving a barium enema;

(f) modifying the usual barium enema solution to make it more dilute;

(g) remembering (if you give the barium enema) not to put in or attempt to put in more than the limited bowel can hold.

5 Before and after handling stoma bags and attending to the stoma, you must wash your hands.

Chapter 24

The 10-day rule

Even before the end of a first day's work in a radiodiagnostic department, a student radiographer is likely to learn that ionizing radiations have biological effects. A radiographer exposing a radiograph administers to the patient concerned a 'dose' which is potentially harmful. Consequently, in the course of our work we are as concerned as are radiologists, physicists and clinicians with the restriction of absorbed radiation dose to the minimum required for a necessary radiodiagnostic investigation.

Answering the question 'Is this X-ray examination necessary?' entails a discretionary decision between two risks for the patient concerned: the radiation risk implicit in an X-ray investigation; and the health risk incurred when a doctor is denied the information with which a radiological examination would equip him. Neither radiographers nor patients are expected to answer this question, but it is one which every doctor should ask himself before he writes a requisition for an X-ray examination. As a rule the decision is easy: the value of the investigation is recognized as being far greater than the magnitude of the radiation hazard to the individual concerned, during the course of the examination concerned, provided that the examination is properly conducted. It is a responsibility of the practising radiographer to ensure that practical procedure keeps the absorbed radiation dose as low as is consistent with securing all the diagnostic information available from any radiographic image.

The protection of a child from radiation is acknowledged to be of particular concern simply because, as he is presumed to have more years of life ahead of him than an adult, his potentiality for the late manifestation of radiation damage is greater. This particular concern for the young should be especially oriented to the unborn child: since the fetus is known to be sensitive to radiation, the principle of avoiding the irradiation of a pregnant woman is attractive.

Adherence to this principle led to the formulation of a so-called '10-day rule', following a first recommendation (ICRP No. 6) of the International Commission on Radiological Protection, in 1964, on the irradiation of women of reproductive age (amended in a later report to 'reproductive capacity'). This 'rule' has been widely misunderstood by radiologists and radiographers, upon whom its implementation naturally depends.

The 10-day rule is concerned with those X-ray examinations which involve the inclusion of a woman's uterus within the primary beam: radiography of the pelvis, lumbar spine or abdomen comes readily to mind. Application of the rule requires such examinations to be scheduled to the pre-ovulatory phase of a woman's menstrual cycle, during which pregnancy is deemed to be physiologically impossible and is certainly extremely unlikely to occur; that is, such significant X-ray examinations are to be made only during an interval of 10 days from the onset of the previous menstruation; unless the medical urgency of the examination is of overriding importance, or the woman either has practised 'satisfactory' contraception or has undergone surgical sterilization. In this way the irradiation of a very early fetus may be generally avoided.

A radiodiagnostic department which practises the 10-day rule faces certain difficulties. Such troubles include:

1 a patient's annoyance when an examination is postponed;

2 a patient's embarrassment over discussion of her menstrual history at a crowded reception desk (a common circumstance in many busy departments);

3 a patient's uncertainty (which is not unusual) of the date of her last menstrual period (LMP);
4 a patient's difficulty in understanding and speaking the language of the country in which she is living, because it is not native to her;
5 a failure of some clinicians to complete the section of the X-ray requisition form which may instruct the department to ignore the 10-day rule in particular cases;
6 difficulty in placing re-scheduled examinations in the department's other work load.

However, there is no evidence to date that the irradiation of a very early fetus is either more damaging or less damaging than irradiation of an ovum during the weeks before fertilization. It is further considered that the most significant risk of fetal maldevelopment occurs during a period of about five months from a date of about one month from the prospective mother's last menstruation, the third and fourth months after the onset of the LMP being particularly significant. It is of medico-legal importance that an early pregnancy should be identified.

The crucial question which the patient should answer is: are you—or might you be—pregnant? She is able positively to say 'No' under any of the following circumstances:

1 if she has had no recent sexual intercourse;
2 if reliable contraception is employed;
3 if she has had surgical sterilization or hysterectomy;
4 if she is post-menopausal.

A woman of reproductive age (13–50 years) who cannot say for certain that she is not pregnant should be held to be in a possible early pregnancy until the contrary is shown to be the case.

A discreet and satisfactory method of handling the important question and answer in practice is to include on X-ray—and other similar—requisition forms a box on the lines of:

Pregnant? Yes/No
Radiographer's signature ....

It is a duty of the radiographer to ensure completion of this section of the requisition form before beginning any examination which entails irradiation of the uterus of a woman of child-bearing age. Unless a patient can be positive that she is not pregnant, or unless there is obvious overriding clinical urgency (for instance, a case of a fractured pelvis), before continuing the radiographer should seek medical guidance from the referring clinician or a radiologist. If it is decided that the examination should proceed, a duty of special care is on the radiographer to ensure that absorbed radiation doses are minimal: the speed of the selected imaging system; accurate collimation and direction of the X-ray beam; and the appropriate use and placing of shielding are significant elements in this care.

Chapter 25

General abdominal preparation

The interpretation of radiographs which visualize any abdominal organ may be hindered—or even prevented—when the area of diagnostic concern includes extraneous images; these images arise from the contents (gas and faeces) of the bowel and are entirely fortuitous. An abdominal radiograph taken of the writer, or a reader, at this moment might—or might not—exhibit sufficient intestinal shadowing as significantly to obscure other abdominal detail; no one can tell until the radiograph is examined.

In consequence, it is common radiodiagnostic practice to prepare a patient for abdominal radiography. Such preparation begins a day or two before the X-ray examination and extends to the day of the examination itself. It is planned to:

1 inhibit the production of intestinal gas by the avoidance of gas-producing foods and aerated drinks;

2 reduce faecal contents by means of a low-residue diet and the use of laxatives.

Gas-producing foods: these include carbohydrates, such as fresh bread; vegetables such as parsnips; 'fizzy' soft drinks.

High residue foods: these include green vegetables and bran.

Laxatives which are suitable include: 'Dulcolax' (bisacodyl); lubricant purgatives, such as 'Normax'; natural bulk-forming evacuants, such as 'Isogel'.

It is customary in a radiodiagnostic department to have ready a printed proforma of instructions for abdominal preparation and to issue this to patients making appointments for abdominal investigations: examples include barium meals, intravenous urograms and plain radiographs of the kidneys, ureters and bladder. Since such preparation often varies in detail between different hospitals, readers of this book are advised to become thoroughly familiar with the practice of their own departments. The following is given only as a typical scheme which might be handed to a patient.

Take the laxative supplied at bedtime on the night before the X-ray examination. (Sometimes the second night before an examination is the preferred time.)

Avoid green vegetables and have a light diet on the day before the examination.

To this can be added any instruction which is particular to the investigation concerned: for instance, six hours starvation before attendance for a barium meal. Finally the form should include statements of the place, date and time of the X-ray examination; and any other necessary remarks, such as advice to bring a dressing gown if it is not the hospital's practice to supply one to outpatients.

Ideal abdominal preparation may be difficult to obtain in practice, particularly in the case of an inactive or bedridden patient: intestinal gas readily accumulates when the subject cannot take exercise.

Chapter 26

Barium meal

During a barium meal, a radiological contrast agent (barium sulphate) is introduced to the gastrointestinal tract by mouth.

Preparation of the patient

1 Inform the patient of date, time and place of the appointment.
2 Explain briefly what the examination will be like, including the length of time involved.
3 Instruct the patient regarding diet and use of laxatives prior to examination. Give printed instructions (available in your department) to the patient and the opportunity to read these with you; ask the patient whether his diet is controlled (for instance, because he is diabetic).
The following is an appropriate set of instructions:
1 on the day before the examination have a light diet, especially avoiding green vegetables;
2 two days before the examination take the supplied laxative in accordance with the attached instructions;
3 take no food or drink during the 6 hours preceding the X-ray examination.

Preparations for the procedure

1 Make ready the X-ray room.
2 Arrange the trolley layout with the following:
(a) the chosen suspension of barium sulphate in the right quantity;
(b) paper cups;
(c) drinking straws (flexi-type);
(d) receivers (in case of vomiting);
(e) skin cleanser;
(f) pre-packed sterile swabs;
(g) needles, syringes, filling tubes (pre-packed) for intravenous injection;
(h) drugs to the radiologist's preference;
(i) containers for disposal of used swabs and 'sharps'.
3 Receive the patient, show him where to undress, provide a clean gown and give a reassurance that you will return to him.

After care of the patient

1 The patient may revert to his normal diet on completion of the examination.
2 The patient should take a laxative to accelerate evacuation of the barium sulphate. This laxative preferably is supplied to him at the time; but practice varies in different hospitals.
3 He should be informed of what he has to do next (for example, that he should make another appointment to see the clinical consultant).

Chapter 27

Barium enema

A barium enema is an X-ray examination of the large bowel by the administration of a radiopaque enema (barium sulphate).

Preparation of the patient

1 Inform the patient of date, time and place of the appointment.

2 Explain briefly what the examination will be like, including the length of time involved.

3 Instruct the patient regarding diet and use of laxatives prior to examination; you should determine whether or not he has had surgery. Give printed instructions (available in your department) to the patient and the opportunity to read these with you. The following is an appropriate set of instructions.

On the day before the examination:

(a) take the supplied laxative between 2 p.m. and 4 p.m.;

(b) eat light, fat-free meals;

(c) eat no solid food after taking the medicine;

(d) limit the evening meal to clear soup, jelly (without fruit), black coffee or tea (with sugar if liked), fruit drinks.

On the day of the examination:

(a) have a light breakfast, if the examination is during the morning

(b) have a light lunch if the examination is timed for the afternoon.

Preparations for the procedure

1 Make ready the X-ray room.
2 Arrange the trolley layout with the following:
- (a) rectal catheters of the preferred type;
- (b) a lubricant for the catheter (K-Y jelly);
- (c) an inflator;
- (d) air-bulb syringes (such as Higginson's);
- (e) disposable suction catheters;
- (f) clinical sheets, gauze swabs as required.

3 Ascertain that the lavatory to be used is clean and tidy and that you know where bedpans are available near-by.
4 Receive the patient, show him where to undress, provide a clean gown and give a reassurance that you will return to him.

Care of the patient

1 Check that the patient has removed clothing and is properly ready for the examination.
2 Assist patient to mount the X-ray table; maintain supportive attitude throughout the examination.
3 With discretion, supervise the patient during any visit to the lavatory and when he is dressing.
4 Advise patient on future actions (resumption of normal diet, next appointment etc.).

Chapter 28

Intravenous urogram

Intravenous urography is a method of opacifying the urinary drainage system by the intravenous injection of a radiological contrast agent, which contains iodine.

Preparation of the patient

1 Inform the patient of date, time and place of the appointment.
2 Explain briefly what the examination will be like, including the length of time involved.
3 Give the patient specific instructions about diet, use of laxatives and dehydration. Such instructions should be printed and you should give the patient a chance to read them with you: you must be alert to the possibility of conditions which would contraindicate the issue of the department's usual instructions. The following is typical of instructions which might be given to a patient before intravenous urography:
(a) if you ordinarily take a laxative, you should refrain from this during the 2 days preceding your X-ray examination;
(b) instead take the laxative provided by the hospital, in accordance with attached instructions;
(c) on the day before the examination have a light diet, especially avoiding green vegetables;
(d) take no food or drink for 6 hours before the X-ray examination.

Preparations for the procedure

1 Make ready the X-ray room.
2 Arrange the trolley layout with the following:
(a) *Sterile.*
Syringes, 60 ml, 20 ml, 5 ml, the first two having a side nozzle filling tubes.
'Butterfly' or similar infusion set.
Needles appropriate to the syringes, e.g. nos. 1 and 16.
'Sterets' for skin cleansing, or surgical spirit plus swabs.
(b) *Non-sterile.*
Phials of the contrast agent.
Dressings bowl containing warm water to maintain the contrast agent at blood heat.
Dressings bowl containing cotton wool swabs.
Plaster dressings and roll of narrow adhesive tape.
A pair of scissors.
Tourniquet or sphygmomanometer.
Padded board or sandbag for support of the arm.
A receiver.

3 Receive the patient. If the patient is female and aged between 13 and 50 years, ask her if she is—or might be—pregnant; then complete the appropriate box on the X-ray requisition form, if the form includes one. Unless the patient is certain that she is not pregnant, or there is overriding medical urgency, medical guidance must be obtained before you proceed with the examination.
4 Provide a clean gown and show the patient where to undress and where a lavatory is; the bladder should be emptied immediately before the X-ray examination.

Care of the patient

1 Adopt a supportive demeanour before and during the administration of the contrast agent. The patient may be asked if he knows that he is sensitive to some foods or other allergens (for instance, chicken feathers). This is in order that you may be forewarned of the likelihood of an allergic reaction following the intravascular introduction of a radiological contrast agent; and to allow the doctor who gives the injection to modify his procedure.
2 When the contrast agent has been given, ensure that the patient is not left alone.
3 Be alert to any change in the patient's condition and obtain medical aid if necessary.
4 On completion of the examination, instruct the patient about what he must do next, for instance he may need to make another appointment to see his consultant.

Chapter 29

Oral cholecystogram

Oral cholecystography is an X-ray examination of the gall bladder by means of a contrast agent which contains iodine and is taken by mouth.

Preparation of the patient

1 Inform the patient of date, time and place of the appointment.
2 Explain briefly what the examination will be like, including the probable length of time involved on each day.
3 Instruct the patient regarding his diet and the use of laxatives prior to examination. Give printed instructions (available in your department) to the patient and the opportunity to read these with you. The following is an appropriate set of instructions relating to the exposure of the control radiograph:

(a) two days before the examination take the supplied laxative in accordance with the attached instructions;

(b) during the day before and on the morning of the X-ray examination the diet should be light and contain little fat.

4 When the control radiograph has been taken the patient requires further instructions about diet and the administration of the contrast agent, before he attends (Day 2) for the contrast radiographs; overnight starvation is necessary. The following are important at this stage of the procedure:

(a) provide the patient with the contrast agent, together with clear written and verbal instructions about taking it;

(b) before instructing him to starve, you must make sure that the patient is not diabetic and receiving insulin (if he is, he should omit the insulin on the morning of Day 2 and must be given an early appointment);

(c) although he should not eat after taking the contrast agent, the patient may be encouraged to drink plenty of water.

5 When poor demonstration of the gall bladder on Day 2 requires a further series of radiographs (Day 3), then renewed instructions about the contrast agent (which may be a different one from the first) and about diet are necessary.

6 The patient should continue on a low-fat diet during the remainder of Day 2 and drink water freely.

Preparations for the procedure

1 Have the X-ray room clean, tidy and in a state of readiness.

2 Have near at hand: the contrast agent(s) in use in the department; a supply of any artificial fat meal that the department favours; for the latter a supply of paper cups and tissues.

3 Receive the patient, show him where to undress, provide a clean gown and reassure him that you will return for his examination.

Care of the patient

1 Ensure that the patient has full explanations during the 2 to 3 days of the examination.

2 On completion of the procedure, advise the patient that he may revert to his usual diet.

3 Inform the patient of his next move (for instance, he may have to make another appointment to see the clinical consultant).

Chapter 30

Intravenous cholangiography

Intravenous cholangiography may be indicated when oral cholecystography has had indefinite results, or for a patient whose symptoms persist after cholecystectomy. When intravenous cholangiography follows the oral procedure, an interval of at least a week between the two examinations is usually recommended.

Preparation of the patient

1 Inform the patient of the date, time and place of the appointment.

2 Explain briefly what the examination will be like, including the length of time involved.

3 Give the patient specific instructions on his preparation and make sure that he understands these. This is best achieved by issuing printed information and allowing the patient time to read this with you. Practice often varies but a typical preparation would put the patient on a light, low-fat diet on the day before the examination and propose a fat-free breakfast on the morning of the examination itself.

Preparations for the procedure

1 Have the X-ray room clean, tidy and ready.

2 Arrange the trolley layout with the following:

(a) *Sterile.*
A 'butterfly' or similar infusion set.
'Sterets' for skin cleansing.
One 5 ml syringe.
No. 16 needles, or similar, for the above syringe.

(b) *Non-sterile.*
A bottle of 'Biligram'.
Water in a dressings bowl to warm the contrast agent.
A bowl containing cotton wool swabs.
A few small plaster dressings for the skin wound.
A roll of narrow adhesive tape.
A pair of scissors.
A tourniquet or sphygmomanometer, or both.
A small sandbag or padded board for support of the arm.
A receiver in case of vomiting.

A dripstand from which to suspend the bottle of contrast agent during the procedure also should be on hand.

3 Receive the patient. If the patient is female and of reproductive age (13 to 50 years), ask her whether she is or might be pregnant; complete the appropriate box on the X-ray form if the form includes one. Unless the patient is certain that she is not pregnant, or you know that her case is of overriding medical urgency, you must obtain medical guidance before you proceed with the investigation.

4 Provide a clean gown and show the patient where to undress, giving the reassurance that you will return.

Care of the patient

1 Adopt a supportive manner before and during the administration of the contrast agent. The patient may be asked if he knows that he is sensitive to some foods or other allergens (such as chicken feathers). If he answers affirmatively this indicates his greater likelihood to suffer an allergic reaction following the intravascular introduction of a radiological contrast agent; and allows the doctor who makes the injection to modify his procedure.

2 Ensure that the patient is not left alone. Be alert to any change in his condition and from time to time check that the infusion of the contrast agent is occurring correctly.

3 On completion of the infusion, withdraw the intravenous needle; use a cotton wool swab to apply pressure to the puncture wound for a moment or two; apply an adhesive dressing.

4 When the examination is concluded, advise the patient on what he must do next.

Chapter 31

Bronchography

Bronchography entails the introduction of a contrast agent to the respiratory tract and requires a high degree of cooperation from a patient. The procedure's main applications are to the diagnosis and treatment of bronchiectasis; both the decline in the incidence of this disease and the development of other imaging techniques have reduced the frequency with which bronchography is performed.

Preparation of the patient

1 Inform the patient of the date, time and place of his appointment.
2 Explain briefly what the examination will be like and give an estimate of how long it will take.
3 Ensure that the patient has clear instructions regarding what he must do before attending for his X-ray examination. Practice varies and preparation may include visits to the physiotherapy department for postural drainage of the lungs; it is certain to include an order to take nothing by mouth for 6 hours before bronchography.

Preparations for the procedure

1 Have the X-ray room clean, tidy and in a state of readiness. Television fluoroscopy may be used.

2 Prepare the trolley. Introduction of the contrast agent may be effected through a nasal catheter or through a short needle which has penetrated the cricothyroid membrane in the throat. Obviously, the method in use by the operator concerned influences what must be made ready. The trolley described below is for a transcricoid injection.

(a) *Sterile.*

One 20 ml syringe for the contrast agent: it should have finger grips, a screw cap and a bayonet junction for the needle.

One 2 ml syringe.

One 5 ml syringe.

Needles for the small syringes, which are for use during anaesthesia of the skin and trachea.

Two short wide-bore needles for injection of the contrast agent; alternatively a special trocar and cannula may be provided.

One pair of dissecting forceps.

One gallipot.

Two small dressing bowls.

A pack containing gauze swabs and a dressing towel.

(b) *Non-sterile.*

Local anaesthetic, for example xylocaine hydrochloride 2 per cent.

The contrast agent, for example 'Dionosil Oily'.

A skin cleanser.

Zinc oxide strapping or small prepared dressings.

A pair of scissors.

A receiver for soiled swabs.

3 Ensure that the patient signs a consent form.

Care of the patient

1 Receive the patient and behave supportively throughout the procedure, doing all you can to elicit his cooperation.
2 During the examination the patient almost certainly will attempt to cough but must be discouraged from doing so; in these circumstances your attitude should be calming; it must never be combative.
3 On completion of the examination, the patient must be warned to take nothing by mouth for four hours at least: this is to allow time for the local anaesthetic to disappear.
4 Post-examination care may include further postural drainage and in this case it is necessary to advise the patient of arrangements with the physiotherapy department.
5 The patient—if he is an out-patient—should remain in the X-ray department for half an hour or so and be encouraged to cough up as much of the contrast agent as possible.

Chapter 32

Hysterosalpingography

Hysterosalpingography is an X-ray examination of the uterus and uterine tubes after the introduction of an iodine-containing contrast agent. Its most usual application is to the investigation of female infertility.

Preparation of the patient

1 Receive the patient on arrival, checking particularly that she is in the first half of her menstrual cycle.
2 Arrange premedication, if this is the department's practice.
3 Show the patient where to undress, provide a clean gown and the reassurance that you will return to her.

Preparations for the procedure

1 Make ready the X-ray room.
2 Arrange the trolley layout with the following:
(a) *Sterile.*
A Cusco's vaginal speculum.
A sponge-holding forceps.
A vulsellum forceps.
A uterine sound.
Dilators in suitable sizes.

A 10 ml syringe.
A uterine cannula.
Two towels.
Swabs.
A pair of rubber gloves.

(b) *Non-sterile.*
A jar of obstetric cream.
A cleansing lotion for the vaginal area.
Ampoules of the contrast agent.
A mackintosh or clinical sheet.
A box of face masks.

(c) *Additional accessories.*
If the uterine cannula is of the suction type, the vacuum pump associated with it should be on hand on the trolley. A bin for soiled swabs and an examination lamp (such as a standard 'Anglepoise') also are usually required.

Care of the patient

1 Your attitude should be supportive and gentle: these patients are usually in a condition of nervous tension about the examination.
2 Provide a sanitary pad to the patient before she dresses.
3 Seek medical attention for a patient who appears to be in severe pain or is experiencing much bleeding.
4 Advise patient regarding next action (for instance, further appointment at out-patients' clinic).

Chapter 33
Angiography

Although it is used of a group which are often called 'special' radiological procedures, the term *angiography* has broad reference: it implies the radiological visualization of blood vessels, following the introduction of a contrast agent. Student radiographers all recognize—perhaps ruefully—that the blood vessels of the body are numerous. Thus, more informative descriptions are needed, which will establish the task-area of any particular angiographic procedure: such words as cerebral angiogram and renal arteriogram are self-explanatory and—with other similar terms—no doubt are familiar to readers of this text.

Within the limits of a small handbook it is manifestly impossible to run through the whole angiographic scenario. The observations which follow are based on angiography by means of percutaneous puncture of the femoral artery, where it lies superficially in the groin, and the introduction of an arterial catheter at that point. This is a commonly employed approach during many angiographic procedures, since the tip of the catheter may be advanced with careful manipulation from the femoral artery to lie within a remote vessel.

Preparation of the patient

A patient for angiography usually must be admitted and his preparation is unlikely to be the immediate concern of a radiographer. Advice from the X-ray department to ward staff is required in connection with the following aspects of the angiogram.

1 The patient's informed consent must be obtained.

2 Local or general anaesthesia is entailed and appropriate premedication should be arranged by the radiologist or anaesthetist.

3 The patient should take nothing by mouth for 8 hours preceding the X-ray examination.

4 The groin should be shaved.

5 Jewellery and any denture should be removed.

6 The patient should be dressed in a theatre gown (as for surgery) and travel to the X-ray department in his bed.

Preparations for the procedure

1 Have the X-ray room clean, tidy and ready; this includes the preparation of specialized equipment such as an image intensifier system and a rapid film changer.

2 Prepare the trolley with the following items:

(a) *Sterile.*

1 angiogram pack (typically containing 3 towels, 1 ruler, 1 gallipot).
Three 20 ml glass syringes.
A 2-way tap.
A 3-way tap.
A 60 cm connector.
A filler.
Two foil bowls.
A scalpel (no. 15 blade).
A Seldinger arterial needle (18G, 2 7/8).
A guide wire.
A 'head hunter' catheter.
A vessel dilator.

An intravenous giving set.
Gowns and gloves as required.

(b) *Drugs and preparations.*
500 ml saline, 0.9%
Heparin, 500 units.
A skin cleanser.
Local anaesthetic (lignocaine 1% w/v, 5 ml).
Contrast agent (such as 'Niopam 300', 1 × 500 ml bottle).

3 Receive the patient, ensuring that he is not left alone; premedicated, he will not be fully alert nor well coordinated physically.

Care of the patient

Following angiography, care of the patient rests largely with ward staff; but radiographers must expect that such care may be in their hands—even if only for a short time—so long as a patient remains in the X-ray department. A radiographer so placed should act in accordance with the following rules.

1 If a general anaesthetic has been given, the usual observations are mandatory (see p. 36).

2 The site of the arterial puncture must be observed frequently for evidence of external bleeding or haematoma-formation (apparent as a swelling).

3 In the event of either of the above occurrences, apply firm pressure to the puncture site and inform the radiologist at once.

4 If the patient complains of pain in the leg and peripheral pulses cannot be felt, the radiologist must be informed at once.

5 Observations should be made—and records kept—of the pulse rate and blood pressure, every 15 minutes over a period of two hours following angiography. A fall in blood pressure, a rise in pulse rate, or both, requires immediate medical attention.

Depending on the nature of the angiographic examination, further aspects of care may be of importance. For example, when a cerebral angiogram has been performed, neurological observations of the patient are relevant; and after brachial arteriography pain in the arm is medically significant.

Chapter 34

Lymphangiography

Lymphangiography is the procedure for radiological demonstrations of the lymphatic system through the use of a suitable contrast agent. It depends on the introduction of a cannula to a lymph vessel in the foot or hand; since these are very small vessels, the cannulation of one of them is not as easy in practice as it may appear from this page.

Even before any radiograph is taken, lymphangiography includes three surgical stages.

1 A dye is injected subcutaneously in the webs of toes or fingers, depending on the case in question. As this dye is absorbed, the lymph vessels become visible in the superficial tissues.

2 A fine cannula is inserted in a selected vessel, through an incision of the skin, and secured with a stay suture.

3 A suitable radiological contrast agent is injected very slowly by means of an electrically driven infusion pump. A slow injection is essential to avoid rupturing small lymph vessels. This part of the process may take an hour or more.

Preparation of the patient

Admission of the patient is necessary if general anaesthesia is to be used or if there must be any preliminary treatment of an infection or oedema; in these circumstances, the patient's preparation is in the hands of staff on the ward. In many cases, however, lymphangiography is suitably performed under local anaesthesia and can be considered as an out-patient examination. The following observations assume the subject to be an out-patient.

1 Advise the patient of the date, time and place of the appointment, including the periods of time involved; this may be about 4 hours on the first day and about 45 minutes on the second day.

2 The patient may eat and drink normally both before and after the X-ray examination. (This is applicable only when the planned anaesthesia is local; otherwise preliminary starvation is essential.)

Preparations for the procedure

1 Have the X-ray room clean, tidy and ready with injection pump and a spot lamp.

2 Prepare the trolley layouts. This is conveniently done on a plan for two, separately considered trolleys: one of these (trolley A) is needed when the patient's foot or hand is injected with patent blue dye; the other (trolley B) is made ready for cannulation of the revealed lymphatics, introduction of the contrast agent, and suturing of superficial incisions when the examination is over.

TROLLEY A

(a) *Sterile.*

One 5 ml syringe.

Needles: 1 × 21G, 1 × 25G.

A gallipot.

Cotton wool balls.

A large water-repellent sheet.

(b) *Non-sterile.*
Methylated spirit or other skin cleanser, such as chlorhexidine.
Lignocaine 1%.
Patent blue violet (2 ml).
One disposable razor.

TROLLEY B

(a) *Sterile.*
A gallipot.
A foil dressings bowl.
Gauze swabs.
A dental syringe.
A dental needle.
A filler.
A pair of Idris forceps.
Two 20 ml (or 2 × 10 ml) syringes, for use with the infusion pump.
A few 21G × $1\frac{1}{2}$ needles.
Two large water-repellent sheets.
Sutures (elevators for the selected lymph vessels).
Two lymphangiogram sets.
One cut down set.
(b) *Non-sterile.*
Methylated spirit or other skin cleanser.
The contrast agent: for instance 'Lipiodol Ultra Fluid' in 10 ml ampoule.
'Lignostab–A100' (local anaesthetic combined with adrenaline).
'Steristrip'.
Normal saline.

In addition to these trolleys, a suturing layout should be prepared for the conclusion of the examination.

(c) *Suturing layout (sterile).*
One cleansing pack.
One suture set.
Gauze swabs.
Sutures, such as 'Mersilk' W501 4/0, 1.5 metric.

Apart from the trolley layouts already described, there are other items which may be needed: these include an antibiotic powder spray for the small wounds; 'Micropore' or other adhesive tape; and sterile packs of gowns, gloves and face masks. Some operators like also to wear a pair of loupe glasses to enhance visibility of the small structures concerned.

3 Receive the patient, ensuring that he receives proper instructions for undressing and that he signs a form consenting to the procedure.

4 The patient should empty his bladder before the examination.

Care of the patient

1 Ensure that the patient has some understanding of what is to occur. This explanation should embrace:

(a) the various stages of the procedure, including the series of plain radiographs on the following day;

(b) blue colouration of his skin, urine, and possibly vision, for about 3 days afterwards due to gradual dissipation of the injected dye;

(c) that he will occupy the X-ray table for several hours, during which he is attached to infusion equipment and must keep certain limbs still.

2 If premedication is to be given in the X-ray department, ensure that proper arrangements are made for this and that the patient is not subsequently left alone. (A drugged patient is less alert mentally and his physical coordination may be poor.)

3 Following injection of the patent blue dye, a patient in suitable condition may be allowed to walk about for 20–30 minutes, in order to aid the dye's dispersal through the tissues. You must ensure that any such activity is effectively supervised.

4 Be actively supportive to the patient at all times. Once infusion of the contrast agent has begun, maintain checks on the effectiveness of the equipment and the patient's well-being.

5 Following lymphangiography, the limb (or limbs) concerned may be supported with crepe bandaging from toes to knee, or fingers to elbow, as the case may be; and the patient advised to keep it elevated for 24 hours.

6 If a large incision has been made, the patient should avoid using the limb for 3 or 4 days.

7 Patients may be advised not to smoke for 48 hours after lymphangiography.

8 Ensure that the patient knows the time and place of his appointment for the subsequent series of radiographs on the next day.

9 Inform the patient of arrangements for removal of the sutures just inserted. (Usually this is done about a week later, but probably elsewhere than in the X-ray department.)

Chapter 35

Radiculography/myelography

When a radiological contrast agent is introduced to the spinal part of the subarachnoid space and radiographs are taken, the procedure is called *radiculography* or *myelography*: the first implies that the lumbar region of the spine is examined, and often the term *lumbar radiculography* is employed; the expression *myelography* usually means that the investigation includes the thoracic and cervical regions of the vertebral column, although it is also sometimes used more loosely as an 'umbrella' term for contrast examinations of the spinal column.

Most commonly the patient is injected with the contrast agent by means of a lumbar puncture, the needle being introduced as usual between lumbar vertebrae 4 and 5. If he is then tilted on a fluoroscopic/radiographic table, the contrast agent moves along the subarachnoid space under the influence of gravity: when the patient is in a Trendelenburg tilt the contrast agent travels towards the skull; when the patient's heels are lower than his head the contrast agent flows downwards, toward the termination of the subarachnoid space at the level of the lower border of the second sacral segment. In this way, television fluoroscopy results in observation of the full length of the spinal column; radiographs are exposed at intervals and in various projections as need dictates.

Occasionally, for a cervical myelogram, the radiological contrast agent may be introduced directly in the neck, by means of a suboccipital puncture at the level of cervical vertebrae 1–2. This is the more difficult approach and has been found also to be the more likely to incur entry of some of the contrast agent to the cranial part of the subarachnoid space (intracranial spill). This mishap may increase the severity of any side effect for a patient and may spoil the examination if insufficient of the contrast agent remains in the spinal part of the subarachnoid tract.

Radiculography/myelography facilitates the diagnosis of lesions of the spinal cord and of prolapsed intervertebral discs. In the latter case, further information is sometimes obtained from *discography*, an allied procedure during which a radiological contrast agent is directly injected to the nucleus of a suspected disc. A similar technique—that is, the siting of a needle, positioned under fluoroscopic control, within the nucleus of a selected intervertebral disc—can be employed to treat a patient who is known to have a lumbar disc displacement and would otherwise be a candidate for surgical excision: the disc can be destroyed if it is injected with a suitable chemical.

Preparation of the patient

A patient for radiculography/myelography will have been admitted to hospital. Consequently, his immediate preparation for the X-ray examination is the concern of medical and nursing staff, who should be fully informed of the radiologist's needs in this respect. The following points should be noted.

1 Whilst premedication is not usually necessary, the condition of the patient sometimes indicates its use.

2 Ample hydration of the patient is significant in minimizing after-effects. He should be on his normal diet whenever possible and fluid intake encouraged.

3 Informed consent to the examination is to be obtained.

4 Jewellery and any denture are to be removed.

5 Clothing: a theatre gown, open at the back; pants; socks.

6 The patient should be brought to the X-ray department in his bed in a sitting position.

Preparations for the procedure

1 Make ready the X-ray room. Lumbar puncture requires asepsis, since infection entering the cerebrospinal tract is potentially serious. The X-ray table must be prepared as a surgically acceptable environment; a bactericidal spray should be used to clean the surface immediately before the examination.

2 Arrange the trolley layout with the following:

(a) *Sterile.*

Two gallipots.

One 10 ml syringe.

One 5 ml syringe.

Needles: typically, 1 × 21G, $1\frac{1}{2}$; 1 × 23G, 1.

A filler.

A lumbar puncture needle, 22G.

A connector. (A length of tubing about 200 mm in length which is fitted with adaptors and is used to make a link between a loaded syringe and a lumbar puncture needle *in situ*.)

An absorbent towel for surgical draping of the patient; usually this has a longitudinal slit in it for exposure of only the lumbar region of the spine.

A pair of rubber gloves of appropriate size.

Gauze swabs.

(b) *Non-sterile.*

A local anaesthetic, such as Lignocaine 1 per cent.

The contrast agent; for example, 'Omnipaque 180 mg/ml' in 10 ml ampoules.

A skin cleanser, such as 'Hibitane' 0.5 per cent in spirit.

Two specimen bottles (for collection of cerebrospinal fluid,

which will be submitted to laboratory analysis).
Diazepam ('Valium') for injection.
A disposable razor.
Some small adhesive plasters, for sealing of the lumbar puncture wound.

Care of the patient

During and after radiculography/myelography, a radiographer attending a patient should be aware of the following points.

1 For the lumbar puncture the patient must lie prone but later may have to turn to other positions; explain this to him and give sympathetic reassurance.

2 Explain simply the movements of the fluoroscopic/radiographic table and the application and use of supports when he is tilted from the horizontal.

3 Ensure that all patient-supports are in good order and are correctly fitted in respect of both the table and the patient. Maintain constant supervision of the patient's safety and comfort.

4 Manage all movements of the patient carefully. Particularly during cervical myelography, the patient's neck should be maintained in extension, in order to avoid intracranial spill of the contrast agent; extension can be achieved from the prone position if a firm support is placed beneath the patient's chin.

5 When the examination is finished and the patient is transferred to his bed for conveyance from the department to the ward, ensure that the back rest is adjusted so that he sits upright.

6 On the patient's return to the ward, elevation of the head (about 20 degrees) is usually maintained for a further 12–24 hours of bedrest. However, some radiologists consider that patients do just as well if they are allowed to sit out of bed in a chair, so long as unnecessary movement is avoided; they may walk to the lavatory, for instance, but should do so gently.

7 Side effects of radiculography/myelography may be present by the close of the examination or may develop later. Headache is the most common of these; but nausea and vomiting, leg pain and leg parathesia have been experienced, severally or together, by a few patients. Occasionally convulsive seizures have occurred; and in some neurological institutes anti-convulsant therapy may be given as a prelude to cervical myelography. Although modern contrast agents are well tolerated, the occurrence of intracranial spill has been a suspected adverse influence on the severity of side effects: radiographers involved in assisting patients to move can do no harm if they keep this thought in mind.

Chapter 36

CT scans

Computed tomography (CT) is no different from other X-ray investigations in the respect that a patient's needs, preparation and care are significantly affected by the nature of the region to be examined and by his condition. For instance, CT scans of the chest and limbs require no particular preparation of the patient; and a patient for a head scan may not be fully conscious and may have multiple injuries which must influence his general handling.

In the confines of our present simple approach to patient-care for and during CT, the following points may be helpful to the reader.

1 If the patient is in a state to understand you, he should be told of the length of time entailed by the procedure, forewarned of the movements of the equipment, and reassured that he will be continuously within your sight from the control room.

2 Brain scans do not require particular preparation, though a restless, confused or agitated patient may need to be sedated before coming to the department, since immobility of the subject during the examination is essential. A child older than 18 months to 2 years, who does not co-operate, may have to be admitted to hospital and examined under general anaesthesia.

3 If the scan is of an abdominal organ, preparation of the patient is likely to include the following:

(a) avoidance of gas-producing foods (see Chapter 25) for two days beforehand;

(b) avoidance of laxatives during the same period, other than any issued by the department;

(c) administration of a bulk-forming bowel evacuant (such as 'Isogel') after breakfast on the morning before and again on the morning of the CT examination (if the patient attends as an out-patient he must receive clear directions for taking the aperient).

4 In the case of an abdominal scan, a patient's final preparation (on arrival in the department) may include giving him an injection of an anti-cholinergic drug (a muscle relaxant) such as 'Buscopan'. Its purpose is to facilitate the CT examination by reducing the gut's motility for a while. After effects, usually mild, which a patient may notice, and of which he should be warned, include:

(a) dryness of the mouth;

(b) tachycardia;

(c) loss of visual accomodation. (The possibility of blurred vision precludes car-driving for some hours.)

'Buscopan' is contra-indicated for a patient who suffers from any of the following:

(a) glaucoma;

(b) prostatic enlargement;

(c) a known sensitivity to anti-cholinergic drugs.

5 Radiological contrast agents are often used to enhance the diagnostic virtues of CT images. For instance, 'Gastrografin' (6 ml), taken orally about $1\frac{1}{2}$ hours before the examination, facilitates identification of various loops of bowel when the abdomen is scanned. Many CT scans entail an intravenous injection of one of the water-soluble, non-ionic organic iodine compounds, such as 'Omnipaque' (iohexol). In these circumstances the usual precautions in case of the occurrence of an adverse reaction should be taken (see Chapter 17).

Chapter 37

Medical ultrasound

Medical ultrasound has merited a place in this book. Though they are not an application of X-rays, these investigations are widely undertaken in radiodiagnostic departments; many radiographers now take further training and become skilled in the uses of medical sonar.

However, a reader of this chapter who supposes a mystique of patient-care during ultrasound examinations would be mistaken: in general they need little preparation, are very easy for the patient, and have no aftermath or side effect.

We all know what we mean by an *echo*: scientifically, it is the reflection of a sound wave by an obstacle. The medical use of ultrasound (sound of a frequency too high to be audible by humans) depends on differing reflections of a sonic beam by the targets (body tissue and organs) at which it is aimed. The sonic energy of these reflections may be easily converted to electrical energy and the impulses displayed on the screen of an oscilloscope, giving us our familiar diagnostic images.

A sonar examination is simple and the stress or inconvenience for the patient concerned is minimal. There is little to consider in regard to his care; but we should remember that a simple procedure warrants as much care as does an elaborate one. The following points may be noted.

1 In preparation, if the examination is of an abdominal organ, the patient usually is instructed to:

(a) follow the same regime of preparation as for abdominal radiography (see Chapter 25);
(b) omit food and such drinks as tea, coffee, and alcohol, on the morning of the examination;
(c) drink two glasses of orange juice or water on the morning of the examination;
(d) avoid (if possible) emptying the bladder just before the examination. (In gynaecological examinations particularly, a full bladder, being transonic, is a helpful 'landmark'.)

2 Depending on the examination concerned, a patient may need the usual provisions of privacy and a suitable X-ray gown, so that he may undress.

3 An 'ultrasound trolley' needs to contain:

(a) a coupling gel (usually provided in a handy tube), which the sonographer will use on the patient's skin to maintain contact between it and the sonar probe;
(b) a box of tissues;
(c) a place for the disposal of the tissues.

4 Reassurance and guidance of the patient are as necessary here as during an X-ray examination.

Chapter 38

Radionuclide imaging

Radionuclide imaging is a technique of investigation in which radioactive substances are introduced into the body and a subsequent study is made of the radiation which the administered radionuclide emits from the site of the organ or tissue which is being investigated. The technique comprises the following procedures.

1 The administration to the patient of a suitable radiopharmaceutical. This is most often done by intravenous injection but in some cases the agent is given orally. Side effects are rare.

2 The use of imaging equipment which functions through detecting the radiations emitted from the disintegrating radionuclide. The instrument most commonly used is the gamma camera.

3 The observance of routine procedures for radiation protection.

4 Care of the patient during the whole examination.

The clinical applications of radionuclide imaging are based on the following points.

1 The images obtained are related to the functioning of organs and they may not well display anatomical detail.

2 This method of examination is non-invasive.

3 Radionuclide imaging is a relatively safe form of investigation. The radiation hazard to the patient is slight since most of the examinations involve only small doses of absorbed radiation.

4 The patient finds the examination relatively easy to accept since it is painless, there are few uncomfortable sensations or experiences and co-operation is easy for him.

5 Where the clinical problem is one of disturbed function, radionuclide imaging may commend itself as the simplest and least risky way of diagnosing the lesion which is present.

In the general care of the patient during radionuclide imaging the following points are to be considered.

1 The patient often requires no special preparation.

2 You must warn the patient that the examination can take some time and may require more than one attendance.

For example, in a renogram to investigate renal failure, imaging is done throughout the first 30 minutes at least after the injection of the radionuclide. Then further examinations may be made at intervals which begin at 60 minutes after the injection and may follow at longer intervals up to 24 hours. In cholescintigraphy (imaging to display the gall bladder) the agent is given to a fasting patient (4 hours fasting). The first image is obtained between 1 minute and 3 minutes after the injection of the radionuclide. Later imaging is done at 10–15 minute intervals up to about 60 minutes after the injection, at which time the gall bladder should be visualized if it is normal. If it is not seen then, further delayed images should be made up to 4 hours and on to 24 hours in a jaundiced patient. Because of the length of time that may be involved the patient must be given details as to the programme in front of him.

3 The patient needs reassurance and encouragement. The gamma camera is an intimidating piece of equipment and it is understandable that a patient may feel nervous as he lies beneath it with the notion that it may descend and crush him. He should not be left alone to contemplate this alarming possibility. You should remain in reasonable proximity as long as he is on the examination couch: it is inadvisable for you to stay close by his side throughout the entire period in view of the fact that he has a source of radioactivity within his body and you may have the care of many such patients during your working day. However, you must not treat him as if his condition represented great danger to you (it does not) and you must talk to him encouragingly as to the progress of the examination which is being made. Parents may safely stay with a child during the whole procedure. Obviously when the intervals between the imaging are a matter of hours the patient may be allowed to leave the examination couch and the room.

4 It may be important to tell the patient to take plenty of fluids. This instruction is to ensure the production of a full flow of urine to eliminate the radionuclide by excretion from the body after the examination is complete.

5 For any procedure you must strictly observe the practices in radiation protection which your department stipulates.

6 You must meticulously apply all techniques for the preservation of asepsis and sterility and for the giving of intravenous injections where they are applicable to the procedure that you are undertaking.

Index

Abdominal bracing 5
Abdominal preparation 90
Accident(s) 38–41
  dangerous occurrences 38, 39
  fatal 39
  first aid *see* First aid
  Health and Safety at Work Act 39
  major injury 39
  reporting (recording) 38, 40
  statutory regulations 39
Administration of drugs 8
Air-bulb syringe 95
Allergy (Allergic effect) 45
Anaesthesia *see* General anaesthesia
Angiography 109–12
Anti-cholinergic drug 124
Artificial ventilation *see* First aid, resuscitation
Asphyxia 47, 52–4

Barium
  catheter *see* Catheter, rectal
  enema 94–5
  meal 92–3
  sulphate 92, 94
Bedpan, giving 10
'Biligram' 102
Bisacodyl ('Dulcolax') 90
Blood pressure
  diastolic 19
  recording 18
  systolic 19
Bronchography 104–6
Burns *see* First aid, burns and scalds
'Buscopan' 124
Butterfly infusion set 29, 97, 102
Butterfly needle 29–30

Cannula
  bronchography 105
  filling (filler) 28, 93, 115, 120
  uterine 108
Cardiac arrest 47, 48–52
Catheter
  'head hunter' 110
  rectal 95
  suction 81–2
Cervical myelography 118
Cholangiography, intravenous 101–3
Cholecystogram, oral 99–100
Cholescintigraphy 128
Clinical thermometer 15–16
Closed fracture 70
Colostomy (Ileostomy) 84–5
  care of patient 85
  stoma bag 85
Coma (Comatose) *see* Consciousness, levels; Consciousness, loss; Diabetic coma; Insulin, coma
Comminuted fracture 70
Complicated fracture 70

Compound fracture 70
Computed tomography *see* Scan(s) CT
Consciousness
  causes of loss 60–7
  levels 80
  loss 59–67
  loss in diabetes mellitus 62
Contrast agent(s) 92, 94, 97, 99, 105, 108, 111, 115, 118, 119, 121, 124
  reactions to 44–5, 119
Controlled drugs (CD) 7
CT scan *see* Scan(s) CT
Coupling gel 126

Dangerous occurrences 38, 39
Diabetes mellitus 62
Diabetic coma 62–3
Diabetic patient 62, 92
Diastolic blood pressure 19
Diazepam ('Valium') 121
'Dionosil Oily' 105
Discography 119
Dressing, sterile 24–7
Drugs
  administration 8
  anti-cholinergic 124
  categorization 7
  controlled 7
  general sales list (GSL) 7
  pharmacy medicines (P) 7
  prescription only medicines (POM) 7
  safe routines 9
  use 7–9
'Dulcolax' (Bisacodyl) 90

Electrical injury 68–9
Emergencies
  equipment for 45–6
  radiological 44 *et seq.*
  resuscitation procedures 45 *et seq.*
Epilepsy 64–6
Enema
  barium 94–5
  giving 20–1
  pack 20–1
External chest compression *see* First Aid, resuscitation

Filling cannula (Filler) 28, 93, 115, 120
Fainting attack 66–7
Fatal accidents 39
Fire
  actions 42–3
  fighting 43
  smoke 42
First aid
  asphyxia 47, 52–4
  broken glass wound 72–3
  burns and scalds 71–2
  cardiac arrest 47, 48–52
  electrical injury 68–9
  epileptic attack 64–6
  fainting attack 66–7
  fractures 69–71
  haemorrhage 47, 54–6
  insulin coma 63
  loss of consciousness 59–67
  objectives 47
  respiratory arrest 47, 48–52
  responsibilities 47
  resuscitation 48–52
  shock 56–9
Fractures
  first aid 69–71
  signs 69–70
  types 70

Gamma camera 127–8
'Gastrografin' 124
General anaesthesia, care of patient 35–7
  induction 36
  observations 36
  termination 36
Glass wounds 72–3

Greenstick fracture 70
GSL drugs *see* Drugs, general sales list (GSL)

Haemorrhage 47, 54–6
Health and Safety at Work Act 39
'Hibitane' 120
Hyperglycaemia 62
Hypoglycaemia 62
Hysterosalpingography 107–8

ICRP (International Commission on Radiological Protection) 87
Identity of patient 1
Ileostomy *see* Colostomy/ Illeostomy
Infectious patient
  ward 74–5
  X-ray department 76–7
Insulin
  coma 63
  functions 62
International Commission on Radiological Protection (IRCP) 87
Intravenous cholangiography 101–3
Intravenous giving set 111
Intravenous injection, assisting 28–31
Intravenous urogram (IVP) 96–7
Iohexol ('Omnipaque') 121, 124
'Isogel' 90, 124

Laxatives 90–1
Laying up a sterile trolley 22–3
Lifting patients 3–6
Lignocaine 111, 115, 120
'Lignostab' 115
'Lipiodol Ultra Fluid' 115
Lumbar radiculography *see* Radiculography/Myelography

Major injury
  accident(s) 39
Medical ultrasound 125–6
Mouth to mouth ventilation *see* First aid, resuscitation
Moving patients 3–6
Myelography *see* Radiculography/Myelography

Needle(s)
  bronchography 105
  butterfly 29–30
  dental 115
  intravenous 93, 97
  lumbar puncture 121
  Seldinger arterial 110
'Niopam' 111
'Normax' 90
No touch technique 22–3

'Omnipaque' (Iohexol) 121, 124
Open fractures 70
Oral cholecystogram 99–100
Oxygen administration
  cylinder 32–4
  incubator 32
  intranasal tubes 32
  mask 32, 33, 34
  observations 34
  radiographer's responsibilities 33–4
  risks 33
  tent 32
  use 32–4

Pack
  enema 20–1
  sterile 25
Patient
  colostomy 84–5
  diabetic 62, 92
  first contact with 1–2
  identification 1

ileostomy 84–5
infectious *see* Infectious patient
lifting 3–6
tracheostomy 78 *et seq.*
Pharmacy medicines (P) 7
POM drug(s) 7
Pregnancy, radiation risks in 86 *et seq.*
Prescription only medicines (POM) 7
Pressure point(s) 56, 57
Pulse
observations 14
radial 13–14
taking 13–14
Purgative(s) *see* Laxative(s)

Radial pulse 13–14
Radiculography/Myelography 118–22
Radiological contrast agent *see* Contrast agent(s)
Radionuclide imaging 127–9
Reaction(s) to contrast agents 44–5, 119
Reception of patient 1–2
Recording (Reporting) accidents 38–40
Recovery position 61, 66
Rectal catheter 95
Renogram 128
Respiration, counting 17
Respiratory arrest *see* First aid, respiratory arrest
Resuscitation *see* Emergencies, resuscitation procedures *and* First aid, resuscitation

Scalds *see* First aid, burns and scalds
Scan(s),
CT
abdomen 123–4
brain (head) 123
chest 123
contrast agent(s) 124
limbs 123
ultrasonic *see* Ultrasound, medical
Shock *see* First aid, shock
Simple fracture 70
Sonar *see* Ultrasound, medical
Sphygmomanometer 18–19, 28, 30
Sterile
dressing 24–7
pack 25
procedure(s) 22–3, 24–7, 28–31, 129
trolley 22–3
Stethoscope 18–19
Stoma bag 85
Stupor (Stuporous) *see* Consciousness, levels
Suction apparatus *see* Tracheostomy, suction procedure
Suturing layout 116
Syringe(s)
air-bulb (Higginsons) 95
angiography 110
bronchography 105
intravenous injection 97
lymphangiography 115
Systolic blood pressure 19

Temperature
normal 15
taking 15–16
Ten-day rule 86 *et seq.*
Thermometer, clinical 15–16
Tracheobronchial suction *see* Tracheostomy, suction procedure
Tracheostomy,
care of patient 78–9
suction procedure 80–3
tube 78, 79, 81
Trendelenburg tilt 118

Trolley,
  angiography 110–11
  barium enema 95
  barium meal 93
  bronchography 105
  hysterosalpingography 107–8
  intravenous cholangiography 102
  intravenous urogram (IVP) 97
  lymphangiography 114–16
  myelography *see* radiculography *below*
  radiculography 120–1
  sterile 22–3
  ultrasound 126

Ultrasound, medical 125–6
Unconscious patient 60–1
Urinal, giving 11–12
Uterosalpingography *see* Hysterosalpingography

'Valium' (Diazepam) 121
Ventilation *see* First aid, resuscitation

Xylocaine hydrochloride 105